Food Allergies

How to Eat Safely and Enjoyably

Written for
The American Dietetic Association
by Celide Barnes Koerner, MS, RD
and Anne Muñoz-Furlong

JOHN WILEY & SONS, INC.

New York • Chichester • Weinheim • Brisbane • Singapore • Toronto

ISBN 0-471-34714-0

Printed in the United States of America

10 9 8 7 6 5 4 3 2

Food Allergies

Written for The American Dietetic Association by
Celide Barnes Koerner, MS, RD,
Research Nutrition Manager
General Clinical Research Center
Johns Hopkins Hospital
Baltimore, Maryland

and

Anne Muñoz-Furlong
Founder
The Food Allergy Network
Fairfax, Virginia

The American Dietetic Association Reviewers:
Tiffani Hays, MS, RD, CNSD
Johns Hopkins Hospital
Baltimore, Maryland

Ellen Karlin, MS, RD, FADA
Baltimore, Maryland

Robert Wood, MD
Johns Hopkins Hospital
Baltimore, Maryland

Technical Editors:
Betsy Hornick, MS, RD
Raeanne Sutz Sarazen, RD
The American Dietetic Association
Chicago, Illinois

JOHN WILEY & SONS, INC.
New York • Chichester • Weinheim • Brisbane • Singapore • Toronto

THE AMERICAN DIETETIC ASSOCIATION is the largest group of food and health professionals in the world. As the advocate of the profession, the ADA serves the public by promoting optimal nutrition, health, and well-being.

For expert answers to your nutrition questions, call the ADA/ National Center for Nutrition and Dietetics Hot Line at (900) 225-5267. To listen to recorded messages or obtain a referral to an RD in your area, call (800) 366-1655.

Contents

Introduction

The term food allergy has long been misused to describe a wide variety of adverse reactions to food, including food intolerances, foodborne illnesses, and food aversions. In one survey of American households, over 16 percent of the respondents believed that they had a food allergy. In reality, only 1 to 2 percent of adults and 5 percent of children are truly affected by an allergy to certain foods. Why do so many people believe they are allergic to food? It's easy to attribute an illness or discomfort to something you ate, and symptoms of other types of reactions to food, such as food intolerances or foodborne illness, often mimic the reactions caused by a food allergy.

Myths abound about the symptoms, causes, diagnosis, and treatment of food allergies. Problems such as poor behavior, hyperactivity, bad breath, weakened immune system, fatigue, forgetfulness, and depression have been blamed on food allergies. Preservatives, food colorings, and spices are believed by some to be major causes of food allergic reactions. Many unproven diagnostic and treatment measures have also been suggested, including rotation diets, vitamin extracts, and bee pollen.

The misinformation lives on through old wives tales, supermarket tabloids, popular books, and misdrawn conclusions. It is fueled by sensational stories of magical cures, lack of information about where to go for accurate diagnoses, and a misunderstanding about what a food allergy is.

This book will help you separate fact from fiction. Chapter 1 describes the different types of adverse reactions to food. It also covers the types of foods that typically cause reactions and common symptoms, and provides answers to common questions about food allergies.

In Chapter 2, you'll learn about the procedures used to diagnose food allergies. Both proven and unproven methods of allergy testing are discussed. You can also read about other types of allergic reactions to foods. Perhaps most importantly, you'll learn how to find qualified professionals, an allergist and a registered dietitian, who can properly diagnose and treat your food allergies. Current food allergy research strategies and goals wrap up this important chapter.

Chapter 3 is devoted to children and food allergies. You'll learn how you may be able to delay or prevent food allergies in your children. Topics such as the role of breastfeeding and how and when to introduce solid foods are covered. You'll receive valuable strategies for managing food allergies in children, including monitoring your child's growth, ensuring that your child's nutrient needs are being met on a restricted diet, and feeding the finicky eater.

Chapter 4 provides detailed instructions for managing the most common food allergies. For instance, you will learn how to read labels and spot terms that provide clues to whether an offending food is an ingredient. Special concerns for certain types of allergies are addressed, and you'll learn how to substitute other foods to ensure a well balanced, nutritious diet.

Chapter 5 offers day-to-day strategies for coping with food allergies. You'll discover tips for avoiding cross contamination at home, grocery stores, and restaurants; making special occasions, such as vacations and eating away from home, manageable; and making an emergency action plan. Current food labeling rules and practices as well as food industry initiatives are also included to help you better understand how the food industry works.

In the appendix, you'll find a sample food diary to get you started in tracking your diet and possible reactions to food. Sample menus free of the common causes of food allergies—milk, eggs, wheat, soy, peanut, fish, shellfish, and tree nuts—are provided for use during a trial elimination diet. If you have a confirmed allergy, you'll want to try some of the easy-to-make, allergy-free recipes. Sources of additional information—from how to find qualified doctors and registered dietitians in your area to nonprofit organizations and mail order specialty food companies—that may be of help are also provided. The glossary of common allergy terms will enable you to better communicate with your doctor. Recommended readings provide additional sources of information and guidance.

Chapter One

Sensitive to Food?

HAVE YOU EVER experienced a queasy stomach or diarrhea after eating and wondered if you were allergic to something you ate? Adverse reactions to food can be caused by an allergy, intolerance to certain food components, microorganisms that cause foodborne illness, or even a psychological aversion. These reactions are classified as either a food allergy or a food intolerance based on the type of reaction that occurs.

Food Allergy

A food allergy, sometimes called a food hypersensitivity, is an abnormal response by the immune system to a harmless food protein that your body mistakenly identifies as a harmful invader. In its role to protect your body, the immune system produces antibodies against that food. When the food, referred to as an allergen, is eaten again, histamine and other chemicals are released, triggering allergy symptoms.

Symptoms of a Food Allergy

An allergic reaction to food can involve the skin, respiratory tract, and digestive tract:

Skin reactions
➤ swelling of the lips, tongue, and face
➤ itchy eyes
➤ hives
➤ rash (eczema)

Respiratory tract reactions
- ➤ itching and/or tightness in the throat
- ➤ shortness of breath
- ➤ dry or raspy cough
- ➤ runny nose
- ➤ wheezing (asthma)

Digestive tract reactions
- ➤ abdominal pain
- ➤ nausea
- ➤ vomiting
- ➤ diarrhea

The symptoms of a food allergy usually occur within minutes or up to two hours after the food is eaten. The severity of the reaction depends on a number of factors, including how allergic you are and how much of the food you ate. Keep in mind, however, that these common symptoms are not caused solely by food allergies; they can have a multitude of causes besides food allergies. If you experience any of these symptoms after eating certain foods, let your doctor know about it.

Are food allergies increasing?

Food allergies seem to be more prevalent than ever before. Peanut allergy appears to be the leading cause for this increase. No one knows why we are seeing an increase in food allergy. Some believe that better health care is simply resulting in increased reporting of the problem and that rates are not actually increasing. Others believe that the early introduction and frequent exposure to certain foods may be increasing the incidence of food allergy.

Food Intolerance

A food intolerance is an adverse reaction to food that does not involve the immune system. A common example is lactose intolerance, a condition caused by a shortage of the digestive enzyme lactase used to break down the sugar in milk, which is called lactose. If you are lactose intolerant, you may experience symptoms such as gas, bloating, and abdominal pain within several hours after eating milk or milk-containing foods. While people with a food allergy must completely avoid an offending food, people with food intolerance can often eat some of the offending food without experiencing symptoms.

Life-Threatening Reactions

In some cases, the allergic reaction is severe and can be life-threatening. The reaction can include numerous symptoms, such as those described previously, in addition to a drop in blood pressure, unconsciousness, and even death if untreated. This severe type of reaction is called anaphylaxis, also known as anaphylactic shock, and can produce symptoms in as little as a few seconds or may develop over several hours. It can be caused by a wide variety of agents, including food, medications (such as penicillin), insect stings (including fire ants), and latex allergy.

While any food can trigger anaphylaxis in those who are susceptible, the most common culprits are peanuts, tree nuts, fish, shellfish, and eggs. People who have both asthma and food allergies appear to be at increased risk for an anaphylactic reaction. Experts believe that the leading cause of fatal anaphylaxis is food allergy. Chapter 5 includes a sample emergency plan for dealing with serious reactions.

Are food allergies hereditary?

A family history of allergies of any type may make you more susceptible to developing food allergies. Although you are not destined to have food allergies, your risk is greater than those without a family history of allergies. Repeated exposure to the major allergens at an early age may sensitize those who are susceptible. See Chapter 3 for more details.

Offending Foods

The foods that account for 90 percent of the allergic reactions in children are milk, eggs, peanuts, tree nuts (such as pecans, walnuts, almonds, and cashews), soy, and wheat. Most children outgrow their food allergies. However, an allergy to peanuts or tree nuts is seldom outgrown. In adults, the most common causes of food allergies are peanuts, tree nuts, fish, and shellfish (including shrimp, crab, and lobster). Unfortunately, these are also the foods most likely to cause severe reactions. Current estimates are between 4 and 8 million Americans are affected by food allergy.

Other Reactions to Foods

Abnormal reactions by other parts of your immune system can cause other types of reactions to food. Six of these disorders are described here.

Gluten-Sensitive Enteropathy (or Celiac Sprue) This disorder is also called gluten intolerance, yet it is not a true food intolerance but an abnormal response of the immune system to gluten. In gluten-sensitive enteropathy, severe damage to the intestinal lining occurs when gluten is eaten. Gluten is a protein found in oats, wheat, rye, and barley. Symptoms of this disorder include abdominal bloating and gas, diarrhea, and weight loss. To confirm the diagnosis of gluten-sensitive enteropathy, an intestinal biopsy is required. Complete avoidance of any food containing oats, wheat, rye, or barley is the only way to treat this disorder and prevent symptoms. This condition is sometimes confused with wheat allergy.

Food-Dependent Exercise-Induced Anaphylaxis This disorder occurs only during exercise. If a person eats certain foods (celery is the most common) and exercises within 2 to 4 hours after eating that food, he or she may experience the following symptoms: itchy skin over the entire body, followed by reddening, swelling, and hives. The reaction may then progress to anaphylaxis. Interestingly, if the person eats the food but does not exercise, or exercises but does not eat the food there is no reaction. The person with this disorder may have a positive prick skin test to the food which causes this reaction. Once the offending food is identified, it is recommended that you avoid exercise for several hours after eating the offending food.

Allergic Eosinophilic Gastroenteritis This disorder results from an infiltration of eosinophils, a type of blood cell that your body makes in response to something that is an allergen. These blood cells accumulate in the lining of your digestive tract and interfere with its normal function. People with this disorder may have nausea and vomiting after eating, chronic abdominal pain, diarrhea, weight loss in adults, or delays in growth and development in children. Diagnosis of this disorder is difficult to confirm, often requiring multiple biopsies of the esophagus, stomach, and intestine.

Food-Induced Enterocolitis Syndrome This syndrome is most often seen in infants and children, but cases have also been reported in adults. It is most commonly caused by cow's milk or soy protein in infants; eggs, wheat, peanuts, nuts, chicken, and turkey in children; and shellfish in adults. Typical symptoms include severe vomiting and diarrhea, which may lead to dehydration. The symptoms develop within 1 to 6 hours after eating the food. This syndrome is diagnosed by a trial elimination diet followed by a food challenge with the eliminated food. Treatment is avoidance of the offending food.

Food-Induced Protocolitis This disorder is seen only in young infants, occurring in the first few months of life. The only symptom of this disorder is bright red blood in the stool, otherwise the infant appears healthy. It is most often caused by cow's milk or soy protein, but has also been associated with eggs, wheat, corn, fish, shellfish, and nuts. Breast fed infants may also develop this disorder because the food proteins are passed through the breast milk. Diagnosis is made by a trial elimination diet, followed by a food challenge with the eliminated food. Treatment is to avoid the offending food. The child is re-challenged at 1 to 3 years of age, at which time most children no longer experience food-induced protocolitis.

Sulfite-Induced Asthma Many adverse reactions have been attributed to sulfites. These reactions include diarrhea, abdominal pain, cramping, nausea, vomiting, hives, itching, rashes, localized swelling, difficulty swallowing, headache, chest pain, feeling faint, loss of consciousness, and changes in body temperatures and heart rate. Yet, in most instances these reactions have not been confirmed using a double blind placebo controlled challenge. This leaves in question whether sulfites or some other agents may be responsible for these symptoms.

For most individuals, sulfites cause no adverse effects, but for a small number of asthmatic patients who have sulfite-induced asthma, sulfites pose a significant risk and can even be life threatening. If you are sulfite sensitive, knowing the source of sulfites in both foods and medications is extremely important.

Sulfites include sulfur dioxide, sulfurous acid, sodium and potassium metabisulfite, sodium and potassium bisulfite, and sodium and potassium sulfite. Sulfurous acid and potassium sulfite are not allowed as additives in foods. In addition to being used in foods and medications, sulfites can also occur naturally in foods.

The Food and Drug Administration (FDA) has taken several actions to protect you by restricting the use of sulfites in foods, but to date there have been no regulations limiting the use of sulfites in medications. Currently, the use of sulfites on fresh fruits and vegetables is prohibited, with the only exception being potatoes.

If you are sulfite sensitive, you should eat only baked potatoes with skin from restaurants and carry-out establishments to avoid potential exposure to sulfites. You will see sulfites listed on the label of all foods which contain significant amounts (>10 parts per million) of sulfites. In addition, the FDA limits the allowable levels of sulfite residues in imported grapes and shrimp. Wine labels will also state if they contain sulfites.

If you or your child is sulfite sensitive, carefully read all labels to avoid an accidental exposure. Here is a partial list of foods containing sulfur dioxide. These foods should be avoided if you are sulfite sensitive.

➤ Dried fruits (excluding dark raisins and prunes)
➤ Dried potatoes
➤ Fruit toppings
➤ Grape juice (listed as white, white sparkling, pink sparkling, red sparkling)
➤ Gravies and sauces
➤ Lemon juice, unfrozen
➤ Lime juice, unfrozen
➤ Maraschino cherries
➤ Molasses
➤ Sauerkraut juice
➤ Wine

Did You Know?

Some fruits and vegetables cross react with pollens, such as ragweed and birch. As a result, many people who are allergic to ragweed may have symptoms—such as itchy mouth, lips, and ears—when they eat watermelon, cantaloupe, honeydew, and bananas. For those allergic to birch tree pollen, eating certain raw fruits and vegetables, such as potatoes, carrots, celery, apples, and kiwi, may cause an allergic reaction. However, if these fruits and vegetables are cooked, no symptoms appear. This common reaction is called Oral Allergy Syndrome.

Chapter Two

Diagnosis and Treatment

IT CAN BE TEMPTING to diagnose and treat your own or your child's food allergy, but suspected food allergies should be evaluated, diagnosed, and treated by a qualified medical professional, such as a board-certified allergist. Self-diagnosis of food allergies can lead to unnecessary restrictions and inadequate nutrient intake, especially in children. In some cases, self-diagnosing a suspected food allergy can delay treatment of a more serious medical problem.

Over the years, several methods of decreasing the body's reaction to food allergens have been proposed, but none have proven successful. Currently, the only proven therapy for food allergies is to completely avoid the offending food. Specific guidelines for avoiding certain foods, depending on the type of allergy, are described in Chapter 4.

Diagnosing a Food Allergy

The first step in the diagnosis of a suspected food allergy is a thorough case history taken by your doctor. You will be asked a series of questions to identify suspected foods and determine what further tests should be done to verify your food allergies. Following the case history, your doctor will perform a thorough physical exam.

Here is a sample set of standard questions. Jot down your answers to these questions before visiting your doctor so you won't need to rely on your memory for this important information.

Does anyone in your family have allergies? If so, who has allergies and to what are they allergic?

What are the typical symptoms of your reaction and what is the order in which each symptom occurs?

Did your reaction cause you any breathing, skin, and/or digestive symptoms?

What was the length of time between your consumption of the suspected food and the first sign of your reaction?

How much food did you eat to trigger the reaction?

Was the food prepared at home? If so, by whom?

Where was the food consumed?

When was your most recent reaction?

Does a similar reaction occur each time you eat that food?

Were you taking any prescription medications or over-the-counter drugs at the time of your reaction?

Have there been any recent changes in your living situation, for example, new pets, remodeling, move to a new home, etc.?

How was your reaction treated? How long did it take for you to resume your normal activities?

The next step in evaluating a suspected food allergy is to conduct various tests to confirm your case history. Your doctor should explain which tests are being performed, how these tests are administered, how long it will take to get the test results, and what information he or she expects to gather from these tests. Examples of tests your doctor may recommend are:

Serum IgE concentration This test requires a small amount of your blood to be drawn. The blood is then checked for how much IgE (immunoglobin E) it contains. High levels of this type of antibody may indicate allergies. This test is a simple screening test and does not provide specific information regarding what is causing your body to release more IgE than normal.

Radioallergosorbent test (RAST) In this test, a sample of your blood is placed on an absorbent disc that contains specific food proteins. If you are allergic to that food, your blood will contain specific antibodies. The disc is then measured for levels of these antibodies. Different laboratories have different systems for numerically ranking the response. In general, high numbers indicate a high level of antibodies, which suggests a possible allergy to that food.

A RAST test is very sensitive. So, if your blood shows no response to a particular food, more than likely you do not have an allergy to that food. However, this test is not very specific, so if your blood reacts to the food, it may or may not mean you are allergic to that specific food. This is called a false positive reaction. One reason for a false positive result may be the similarities between various foods of a food family. For example, if you are highly allergic to peanuts, your blood may also react to other legumes, such as green beans. It is very important to discuss the results of this type of testing with your doctor. The results should be compared with the information from your case history and other testing methods to determine whether the positive results are true or false. Between 50 to 60 percent of positive test results are false positives.

Prick Skin Tests This test involves introducing a solution containing a specific food protein into the top layer of skin using a blunt two-pronged needle or similar device. Approximately 15 minutes after the solution has been administered, the results are read. For the testing of fruits and vegetables, the actual fresh food may be used rather than a solution. Reading the results involves precise measurement of the skin reaction. Positive results are indicated by a hive (a raised white bump, usually irregularly shaped) surrounded by an area of increased reddening of the skin.

Any food to which your skin showed a reaction is called a positive result. In general, a large hive is more likely to indicate a true food allergy, but size is not always an accurate predictor. Prick skin tests, like the RAST, can be inaccurate, with 50 to 60 percent of positive test results being false positive. Your test results should be compared with your case history and any other tests to determine which of the results are true positives. If your skin did not react, you are probably not allergic to the test foods.

Double-Blind, Placebo-Controlled Food Challenge (DBPCFC) This testing method is considered to be the gold standard for the diagnosis of a food allergy. In fact, it is so accurate that it is often used to verify the results of other tests. A food challenge has the potential for causing an allergic reaction and should only be performed with proper medical supervision and immediate access to emergency medical services. DBPCFCs are not performed by all allergists, therefore your access to this type of testing may be limited.

The test requires you to eat a safe food (a food that causes you no difficulties) that contains either a specific amount of a suspect food (a food to which you may be allergic) or a placebo food (a food which you eat with no difficulties). You are given the suspect food and the placebo food at separate times and neither you nor your doctor knows which you are receiving.

The food challenge is given in measured doses. Following each dose, you are observed for a period of time for any signs of a reaction. In the absence of symptoms, increasingly larger doses are given. If you show any signs of a reaction, the food challenge will be stopped. Once both the suspect food challenge and the placebo food challenge have been completed, the doctor will be informed as to when each was given. He or she will then discuss your food challenge results. You will be asked to restrict from your diet any foods to which you had a reaction.

Open Challenge In this type of food challenge, you will be asked to eat a suspect food that is not disguised in any way, so you will know what you are eating. Open challenges are used primarily in two situations. The first is as a final confirmation of a negative DBPCFC. If you complete a DBPCFC and show no signs of a reaction, your doctor will then have you eat a standard portion of the suspected food to verify that you are not allergic. An open challenge is also used to test a food that produced a positive RAST or prick skin test, yet, from your history, is not thought to be causing any allergic reactions. Like the DBPCFC, open challenges have the potential risk of causing an allergic reaction and should only be performed with proper medical supervision.

Elimination Diets If you have a strongly positive RAST or prick skin test result, your doctor may recommended a trial elimination diet. This type of elimination diet restricts a particular food or foods for a period of 2 to 4 weeks. If your symptoms improve significantly, your doctor may be convinced that this is a true food allergy and have you avoid that food. If, however, your symptoms do not improve or there is unclear improvement, then food challenges would be recommended to clarify the diagnosis.

The long-term use of an elimination diet should always be verified with a DBPCFC. If you or your child is on an elimination diet, a nutritional assessment should be obtained initially and at least every six months or whenever a food is removed from the diet to ensure adequate energy and nutrient intake. Sample elimination diet menus are provided in Appendix 3.

Unproven Methods of Allergy Testing

Some methods of allergy testing are considered controversial. Be aware that these methods of testing have not been proven to give accurate results.

Cytotoxic Testing (Bryan's Tests) This test combines your blood with a specific food protein. Your blood is then analyzed for how many white blood cells it contains. If the number of white blood cells drops, the test is said to be positive, indicating an allergy. To date, no research studies have been able to substantiate this type of testing in the diagnosis of food allergies.

Sublingual Testing This test consists of placing drops of a solution containing a specific food protein under your tongue. If you show signs of a reaction, a weaker solution of the same food protein is placed under your tongue. This second solution is referred to as the neutralizing dose. You are then told to give yourself a neutralizing dose before eating that food to prevent symptoms of a reaction. This type of testing is not recommended as an effective test or treatment for food allergy.

Intradermal Skin Testing This test involves injecting a solution containing a specific food protein underneath your skin. Your skin is then examined for signs of hives and erythema (increased reddening of the skin), similar to prick skin testing. This type of testing is more invasive because the needle actually pierces your skin. This results in an even higher number of false positives and an increased risk for an allergic reaction to the testing. This test is not recommended for the diagnosis of food allergies.

Subcutaneous Testing This type of testing involves injections of specific amounts of food extract. Individuals showing signs of a reaction are then given a neutralizing dose, which is actually a more dilute injection of the same food extract. This neutralizing dose is the treatment for the reaction. The diluted food extract is then formulated into an oral dose so drops can be placed under the tongue before eating the offending food. This type of testing and treatment is also not recommended.

IgG Testing This test involves drawing a blood sample, which is analyzed for the presence of food-specific IgG (immunoglobulin G) and/or IgG subclass antibodies. Food-specific IgG and IgG subclass antibodies have been found in both allergic and non-allergic people. Experts feel that their production is a normal response to eating foods and that this test is not helpful in the diagnosis of a food allergy.

Treating a Food Allergy Reaction

The only proven therapy for your food allergies is complete avoidance of the specific food. Various medications have been tried, but to date, none have been proven effective in prevention or treatment of food allergies.

While avoiding specific foods to which you are sensitive is the only way to prevent a reaction, you should be familiar with how to treat an allergic reaction should one occur. Your doctor will recommend the best treatment measures for your situation.

Skin Rashes (Eczema) Eczema may be treated with a combination of any of the following techniques:
> ➤ Soaking baths or wet wraps immediately followed by liberally applying petroleum jelly to the skin to seal in the moisture.
> ➤ Antihistamines to relieve the itchiness.
> ➤ Antibiotics to treat any possible skin infections, which can cause the skin to itch and worsen the eczema.

➤ Topical steroids applied to areas of increased irritation.

Breathing Problems Difficulties with your breathing require immediate medical attention. The types of treatments include:
➤ Epinephrine given either by spraying a mist into your lungs or by an injection.
➤ Medications called bronchodilators may be given to help expand the tightened breathing tubes of your lungs.
➤ Steroids may be given through an IV or by mouth to decrease the swelling of your throat and lungs.

Gastrointestinal Problems
➤ Symptoms of abdominal pain, nausea, vomiting, and diarrhea are often initially treated with antihistamines.
➤ If symptoms worsen or include persistent vomiting or diarrhea, an injection of epinephrine and intravenous fluids may be needed.

Anaphylactic Reactions Treatment of an anaphylaxis, a severe allergic reaction, requires immediate action:
➤ At the first sign of an anaphylactic reaction, a shot of epinephrine (EpiPen Jr., EpiPen, or Ana Guard) and a liquid antihistamine (Benadryl or Atarax) should be given.
➤ Call 911 immediately.
➤ It is very important that you get to the nearest hospital or emergency clinic as soon as possible for further treatment. Even after your condition stabilizes you will need to be watched for signs of a second, or biphasic, reaction over the next four to six hours.

Every individual with a food allergy should be warned of the potential for an anaphylactic reaction and be taught the appropriate treatment. You are at increased risk for an anaphylactic reaction if you have both asthma and food allergies or a previous history of an anaphylactic reaction.

Working with Qualified Professionals

How to Find an Allergist

The first step in finding an allergist to help you diagnose and manage your food allergies is to contact either the American Academy or the American College of Allergy, Asthma and Immunology (a Resource Guide is provided in the Appendix) and ask for a list of board certified allergists in your area. Next, contact their offices and inquire as to whether the allergist treats people with food allergies.

Once you find an allergist with an interest in food allergies, ask about what you should expect during your first visit. Discuss the type of testing used to diagnose food allergies and what types of treatments are offered. Ask if there is a registered dietitian associated with the practice. If you are comfortable with the responses, then make arrangements for an appointment. At the conclusion of your first visit, ask yourself if you are comfortable with this doctor. You should feel at ease asking questions and discussing your care. If you don't feel comfortable, your care may be compromised because you will not be sharing important information with your doctor. Look for someone with whom you can be open and work closely with to manage your food allergies.

The Role of the Registered Dietitian

The dietitian's primary role in the treatment of food allergies is to help you learn how to manage your food allergy through diet; in other words, how to completely avoid the offending food.

If your testing confirms a food allergy, a dietitian will guide you in how to begin a food-restricted diet. Information that a dietitian can provide includes:

➤ how to determine if a food contains an ingredient that must be avoided by looking for words or phrases on food labels that indicate the presence of an allergen,

➤ how to appropriately substitute certain foods with other "safe" foods, and

➤ sources of special products or recipes for your specific food allergy.

Together with your dietitian, you will develop a personalized eating plan for a well-balanced and nutritionally complete food restricted diet. If it is not possible to meet nutrient requirements on the restricted diet, your dietitian may recommend a vitamin/ mineral or other supplement specific for your needs.

You may be asked to keep a record of what you have eaten over a 3- to 7-day period. This record can be used to check the quality of your diet and to look for hidden sources of the restricted food. Your dietitian may request to see your diet record before your first visit and periodically at follow-up visits. (See Appendix 1 for a sample diet diary.)

The American Dietetic Association can help you locate a registered dietitian in your area who specializes in food allergy treatment. (See Appendix 5.)

Future Treatments for Food Allergy

Scientists are conducting research that may someday offer methods for preventing allergic reactions. As we learn more about how the immune system functions, ways to alter the body's response to allergens may emerge. Promising research is being conducted in the development of vaccines that would block the body's production of antibodies in response to allergens or prevent the release of histamine. These alternative approaches would have far-reaching implications for preventing serious allergic reactions and increasing the enjoyment and flexibility of food choices for people with food allergies.

Chapter Three
Children and Food Allergies

REST ASSURED, you are not alone if your child has been diagnosed with a food allergy. Estimates are that 1 out of every 20 children is allergic to one or more foods. As a parent, you probably have concerns about how you can minimize your child's chances of developing a food allergy, and if your child is already known to be allergic to one or more foods, how you can provide a safe well-balanced diet that will promote normal growth and development. This chapter provides the guidance you need.

Is Your Child at Risk?
Your child's risk for developing food allergies is partly based on your family's history of allergies. Your family history is considered positive for allergies if at least one parent or child has confirmed food allergies or other types of allergies, such as hay fever, asthma, or eczema. A child born into a family with a positive history has two to three times higher risk for developing food allergies than a child from a family with no history of allergies. This means that nearly 10 to 15 percent of children from allergic families may develop food allergies during the first two years of life.

Another factor in the development of food allergies in children is exposure to certain foods. You can't change your family's history, but you can delay the introduction of the eight major food allergens (cow's milk, egg, soy, peanut, nuts, wheat, fish, and shellfish). Delaying introduction of these foods may prevent, decrease the severity of, or delay the onset of food allergies by allowing your child's immune system to fully develop before it is exposed to these highly allergenic foods.

Breastfeeding

Breastfeeding provides your baby with the best possible start in life for many reasons. Breastfeeding promotes the development of factors that reduce the absorption of food antigens, which cause food allergies, and provides protection from viruses and bacteria that the child's immune system would have to fight. Breast milk also contains fewer foreign proteins than infant formula, thus fewer proteins that the immune system has to decide are safe or harmful. Overall, breastfeeding promotes a faster and more efficient development of an infant's immune system.

Breastfeeding for as little as one month has shown potential benefits in decreasing the incidence of allergies. In general, breastfeeding, whether for one month or twelve, provides the greatest protection against allergies during the first two to three years of life.

Should you restrict your diet while breastfeeding?

The increased incidence of peanut allergy in this country has prompted allergists to recommend the avoidance of peanuts and peanut products for breastfeeding mothers. If you are excluding peanuts from your diet, you should eat a varied diet which includes other legumes, whole grains, and vegetable oils to replace the nutrients found in peanuts. For infants who are at high risk of developing food allergies, other foods may be restricted in the mother's diet. These additional food restrictions should be discussed with your doctor.

Formula Feeding

Always consult with your doctor prior to feeding your baby any new formula. Typically, a milk-based formula which has been extensively hydrolyzed (broken down) is recommended for weaning or supplementing a breastfed food-allergic infant. There are three products currently available with milk protein that is extensively hydrolyzed and recognized as hypoallergenic. These are Nutramigen, Alimentum, and Pregestimil.

Occasionally, an infant will have an allergic reaction to these formulas and a synthetic amino acid based formula will be prescribed. This type of formula is very expensive and is only utilized for infants who are exquisitely allergic to milk. Neocate is currently the only amino acid based infant formula available for this use.

Introducing Solid Foods

The answer to the age-old question, "When should I introduce solid foods?" can vary depending on who you ask. In general, introducing solid foods to babies with confirmed food allergies and those babies with a higher risk of developing allergies should be gradual and conservative.

The following guidelines are intended for babies with a family history of allergies and for babies with confirmed food allergies. Be aware that these guidelines may vary from infant feeding guides found in general parenting books and magazines. Your doctor and dietitian can guide you how and when to gradually introduce solid foods to your baby. Chapter 4 provides additional guidance on choosing and substituting specific foods.

Will my child outgrow a food allergy?

Many children do outgrow their food allergies. However, allergies to peanuts and tree nuts are seldom outgrown. Reintroducing small amounts of an offending food is not recommended because this may actually prolong a food allergy. Your doctor will decide, based on your child's allergy test results, when allergenic foods should be re-introduced, if ever. Any food to which your child has had a confirmed allergic reaction should only be given in a doctor's office where immediate medical attention is available. A food that caused a severe anaphylactic reaction should only be re-introduced with extreme caution.

First Foods and Beyond

In general, solid foods should not be given before your baby is 6 months old. A single grain, iron-fortified cereal is usually recommended as your baby's first food. Baby rice cereal is typically the cereal of choice as a first food for a food-allergic baby. A single grain cereal will only introduce one type of protein. Be sure to read the ingredient statement carefully to check that the cereal is a single grain. Some cereals also contain malt, which is made from barley, and other ingredients. These cereals would expose your child to more than one food protein at a time. Your baby can continue on rice cereal for a month before advancing to other foods.

At about 7 months of age, you can begin introducing vegetables and fruits, starting with orange vegetables. Squash is usually first, followed by sweet potatoes and carrots. Your baby should be given a new food for 5 to 7 days before advancing to the next food. This allows you time to observe your baby for any signs of an allergic reaction.

Once the orange vegetables have been successfully introduced, the diet can be expanded to green vegetables, including spinach, green beans, and peas. Be sure to carefully read the ingredient lists on baby food since some varieties of spinach and peas contain milk products. The best rule of thumb is to stay with the early stage vegetables and fruits, which are packed in water only.

Fruits may be given in any order, but remember to give only single fruits, not fruit mixtures or fruits containing tapioca or food starch. A sample order of introducing fruits may be applesauce, pears, plums, peaches, apricots, pineapple, and banana.

How do I know if my child's diet is providing enough nutrients for growth and development?

One way to determine whether your child is receiving enough nutrients is to monitor growth. It's important to have your child's weight, height, and head circumference measured at regular intervals, usually every six months after their first birthday. Additionally, your child's growth should be checked within one month after any major dietary changes such as additions or restrictions of foods. Your child's growth should be recorded on a standard growth chart where the measurement can be translated to a percentile. The 50th percentile is considered average for each of these measurements. Plotting your child's measurement on a growth chart allows your doctor to monitor changes in your child's growth pattern. If your child's growth slows significantly, further evaluation by your doctor or a registered dietitian is recommended.

By the time you finish introducing vegetables and fruits your baby will be approaching 9 months of age and ready for the introduction of other grains and vegetables. Begin with oats, then corn, white potato, barley, and finally wheat. As before, always read the ingredient label to be sure you are giving a single food and give that new food for 5 to 7 days before advancing to the next one. The next step is to begin adding table foods. You may introduce other vegetables and legumes that your family eats. At one year of age you can also begin to add meats to your child's diet. The order for introducing meats usually begins with lamb, then advances to pork, turkey, chicken, and beef. Continue to introduce new foods gradually and watch for signs of an allergic reaction.

If your child is at risk for developing food allergies, highly allergenic foods, including milk, soy, egg, peanuts, nuts, fish, and shellfish, can be introduced at these times:

➤ At 1 year of age, milk and soy.
➤ At 2 years of age, eggs.
➤ Between 3 and 4 years of age, peanuts, tree nuts, fish, and shellfish.

Signs of an Allergic Reaction in Infants and Young Children

As new foods are introduced to a child's diet, watch for these signs that an allergic reaction may be occurring. Signs are usually evident in your child's skin, breathing, or digestion.

➤ itchy eyes
➤ runny nose
➤ swelling of the lips, tongue, and face
➤ itching and/or tightness in the throat
➤ shortness of breath

- dry or raspy cough
- wheezing (asthma)
- rash (eczema)
- hives
- abdominal pain
- nausea
- vomiting
- diarrhea

Signs of an allergic reaction can occur within minutes or up to 2 hours after your child has eaten. Always let your doctor know if any of these symptoms coincide with the introduction of a new food.

Assessing Your Child's Nutritional Status

A registered dietitian can perform a complete nutritional assessment, which includes assessing your child's weight, height, and head circumference measurements, evaluating blood test results, reviewing your child's growth and development, estimating your child's energy and nutrient requirements, and providing a plan for a nutritionally complete diet.

During the assessment, your dietitian will take a detailed history of your child from birth to the present and ask a series of questions, such as the following:

- What was your child's birth weight, height, and head circumference?
- Did your child have any difficulties at birth?
- Does your child have any special medical problems?
- Is your child on any medications? If so, what are they, how much, and how often are they taken?
- Was your child breast or formula fed? If breastfed, for how long? Did the mother follow any dietary restrictions while nursing?
- If formula fed, what formula or formulas were used and for how long? If the formula was changed, what was the reason for the change?
- When were solid foods introduced? In what order were they introduced (for example, cereals, fruits, vegetables, then meats)?

- Were there any problems with solid foods? If so, list the foods and describe the symptoms which occurred.
- When were table foods introduced?
- Has your child had the following foods and at what age were these first given? Milk, egg, soy, peanut, nuts, wheat, fish, and shellfish
- Has your child been diagnosed with food allergies? If so, how and when were they diagnosed?
- Are you currently restricting any foods from your child's diet? If so, how long have you been restricting these foods?
- What type of doctor is monitoring your child's food allergies?
- What is the doctor's plan for follow-up?
- Has your child ever had an allergic reaction to a food? If so, describe the reaction. What food caused it? How was the reaction treated?
- What percentiles was your child's weight, height, and head circumference at the last doctor's visit? Have the percentiles been consistent? If they have changed, is your doctor concerned?
- Do you have any concerns about your child's weight, height, or head circumference?
- What is your child's bowel movement pattern? Describe the consistency of the stool. Does your child complain of stomachaches? If so, how often and have you been able to associate it with a particular food? How often does your child vomit?
- Describe what your child eats in a typical day. What meats, starches, vegetables, and fruits does your child eat? What does your child drink most often?
- Does your child take any vitamin and mineral supplements? If so, which ones and how often?

The dietitian may also ask you to keep a food diary. In the food diary, you will record everything your child eats and drinks daily. You will also record how the food was prepared, brand names of commercial products, and if you added any condiments, sauces, or toppings to the food. This record is usually kept for 3 to 7 days. A sample diet diary is provided in Appendix 1.

Using a computer program, the dietitian will analyze the diet record. The analysis will provide a summary of your child's intake of calories, protein, carbohydrates, fats, vitamins, and minerals. The dietitian will review this summary and look for any nutrients which may be below daily requirements. These requirements are based on your child's age and sex. Depending on the results, the dietitian may recommend changes in your child's eating pattern. If certain nutrients are lacking due to food restrictions or food dislikes, the dietitian can provide specific suggestions for alternative food choices or appropriate supplements to meet your child's individual needs.

Your child's diet should be periodically assessed thereafter to ensure that the right amounts of nutrients are being provided for growth and development. When foods or food groups are eliminated, it's important that other foods be substituted to provide the missing nutrients. Using the Food Guide Pyramid as a guideline for food choices and emphasizing fresh, unprocessed foods will provide the foundation of a well balanced diet. Meeting special dietary needs and avoiding certain foods is often easiest by cooking from scratch. Homemade foods also allow you to substitute foods with similar nutrient content.

Once your child's diet has been reviewed by the dietitian, you will be given specific recommendations for food, and formula for infants not being breastfed. The best way for your child to get nutrients is from foods. If vitamin and mineral needs cannot be met by diet alone, you will need to discuss the use of a supplement with your dietitian and doctor. Be sure to check the ingredients of your supplement for potential allergens.

Calories. Calorie needs are estimated based on your child's age, weight, activity level, and state of health. The dietitian will calculate your child's calorie, or energy, needs using your child's current weight. Monitoring growth is the best indicator for knowing if your child's energy needs are being met. If your child has eczema, asthma, or any other chronic medical condition, additional calories and nutrients may be required.

Protein. Protein needs, like calories, are based on age and weight. While protein-containing foods are the most common food allergy culprits, restricting one or more protein-containing foods will probably not impact your child's ability to meet protein requirements. Protein is abundant in many different foods, and meeting protein needs is not difficult if a variety of protein sources are included. Primary protein sources include meats, poultry, fish, eggs, and milk products. Vegetables, legumes, nuts, and grain products are also protein sources, but contain smaller amounts than foods derived from animal products.

Protein is composed of units called amino acids. There are two types of amino acids—essential and non-essential. Essential amino acids come only from the foods you eat, whereas non-essential amino acids can come from foods or be made by your body. Foods containing animal products contain all of the essential amino acids your body needs and are considered high quality protein sources. Foods that come from plants do not contain all of the essential amino acids. However, eating several different plant foods, such as legumes and grains (beans and rice) or nuts and grains (peanut butter on bread), at meals and over the course of a day will help to provide all the essential amino acids. A dietitian can check your child's diet for appropriate amounts of both protein and essential amino acids.

Carbohydrate. Carbohydrates are the primary source of fuel for your child's body. At least 50 percent of your child's calories should come from carbohydrates. The best sources of carbohydrates are whole grains, legumes, fresh vegetables, and fruits because these foods not only provide carbohydrates but are also sources of important vitamins and minerals.

Fat. Fat is also an important source of energy for fueling your child's growth and high activity level. Fats are a concentrated source of calories since they contain twice as many calories as equivalent amounts of carbohydrate and protein. This is important because children have a small stomach relative to their large calorie needs. After age 5, about 30 percent of a child's calories should come from fats. The sources of fats include animal products, which provide primarily saturated fats, and plant products, which provide mono- and polyunsaturated fats. A balance of these three types of fats is recommended for a healthy diet.

Vitamins and minerals. There are over 25 essential nutrients which your child's body needs daily. Food restrictions can limit intake of important vitamins and minerals. Some of the key nutrients to focus on in your child's diet are vitamins: A, D, E, B_{12}, B_6, C, pantothenic acid and folate; and minerals: calcium, magnesium, zinc, and copper. The table below lists some food sources of these nutrients.

Nutrient	Food Sources
Vitamin A	Carrots, spinach and other dark-green leafy vegetables, fortified milk and milk substitutes (for example, soy, rice, and potato milk), liver, fish oils, and eggs
Vitamin D	Fortified milk and milk substitutes, fortified cereals
Vitamin E	Vegetable oils, wheat germ, and nuts
Vitamin B_{12}	Meat, poultry, fish, shellfish, and milk products
Vitamin B_6	Chicken, turkey, liver, pork, eggs, whole grain rice, oats and wheat, peanuts and walnuts
Vitamin C	Fruits and vegetables, especially oranges, grapefruit, tangerines, and other citrus fruits, strawberries, tomatoes, broccoli, spinach and other dark-green leafy vegetables, peppers, and potatoes
Pantothenic Acid	Meat, poultry, fish and shellfish products, whole grain rice, corn, wheat, rye, oats, and barley, and legumes, such as peas, beans, lentils, soy, and peanuts
Folate	Spinach and other dark-green leafy vegetables, legumes (for example, peas, beans, lentils, soy, and peanuts), liver, yeast, and fortified foods
Calcium	Milk products, fortified milk substitutes (for example, soy, rice, and potato milks), fortified fruit juice and drinks, and other fortified foods
Magnesium	Whole grain rice, corn, wheat, rye, oats, and barley, legumes (such as peas, beans, lentils, soy, and peanuts), seeds and nuts
Zinc	Meat, poultry, fish and shellfish products, eggs, and whole grain rice, corn, wheat, rye, oats, and barley
Copper	Fish, shellfish, liver, seeds, and nuts

Feeding the Finicky Eater

Handling a toddler or young child on a food-restricted diet can be challenging. Here are some strategies that may help you and your child through any difficult times.

Be creative with your presentation of foods. For example, serve carrot curls instead of carrot sticks by peeling your carrots, then placing the peels in cold water and refrigerating them. As the peels chill, they will curl. This not only makes eating carrots more fun but easier for a toddler who may not want to chew a carrot stick.

Keep foods simple. Casseroles may not be popular with toddlers and young children unless you limit the combination of foods, for example, pasta with tomato sauce; many children prefer foods separated on the plate. This allows the child the pleasure of eating one food at a time.

Serve finger foods. This provides enjoyment from eating foods and provides opportunities for exploring different textures.

Vary the temperature of foods served. Serve vegetables raw with a special dip if your child refuses cooked vegetables. If fresh fruits are refused, serve canned or cooked fruits. For variety, serve frozen fruits, such as banana slices.

Use pureed vegetables, legumes, and fruits to fortify your child's diet. These can add vitamins and minerals to your homemade soups, casseroles, and baked goods without your child knowing it. For example, add pureed pinto beans to a tomato-based soup, or pureed sweet potatoes to apple muffins.

Serve dinner foods at breakfast and vice versa. A baked potato for breakfast is just as healthy as a bowl of cereal. Your child will eat a better diet if you provide access to healthy foods throughout the day. Restricting your growing child's intake to mealtimes only may not provide the calories and nutrients needed.

Ignore food swings—they are usually short-lived. Although you may be bored with making the same foods day in and day out, your child probably is not bored eating them, and more than likely, the diet is nutritionally complete. If, however, you have serious concerns regarding limited food preferences, ask a dietitian to review your child's diet.

Involve your child in preparing foods. Children take pride in the accomplishment of preparing food and may be more willing to eat that food.

Invite other children over at mealtimes. This makes mealtime more festive and pressure from peers often encourages children to try new foods.

How can I be sure that my child will not be served a food that he or she is allergic to when away from home?

Talk to your child about why it is so important to avoid certain foods. Children themselves, even toddlers, can play a role by refusing any food unless it is served by a parent. Role play various situations that may occur so your child is prepared and knows how to handle them. See Chapter 5 for additional strategies.

Chapter Four
Managing Food Allergies

ALTHOUGH ANY FOOD can cause a food allergy, eight foods cause approximately 90 percent of the allergic reactions. This chapter provides basic guidelines on how to manage common food allergies by avoiding the offending foods. Knowing to avoid a certain food may seem straightforward, but it can be challenging when that food is used as an ingredient in many other foods, and when there are many different ingredient terms for that food. It's also important to know what other foods can be substituted to provide an alternative source for the nutrients otherwise found in the offending food.

Learning to read food labels is an essential skill in managing a food allergy. Be aware that food manufacturers may change ingredients and labels without warning, so you should check the food label each time you buy a food. Foods without an ingredient listing should be avoided, especially if there is any possibility that an offending food might be included. If there are terms on the label that you do not understand, call the manufacturer. The best rule of thumb is, "When in doubt, don't eat it."

Milk Allergy
Milk is a common allergy-causing food in young children. If you or your child has been diagnosed with a milk allergy, you must remove all milk and milk by-products from the diet. This includes yogurt, butter, most margarines, cheese, cream, and milk.

Milk is an important source of calcium, vitamin A, vitamin D, riboflavin, pantothenic acid, and phosphorus. Enriched soy, potato, or rice milk beverages are good alternative sources of calcium, vitamin A, and vitamin D. These enriched drinks can also be used as a substitute for milk in recipes. Calcium can also be provided by tofu made with calcium, calcium-fortified orange juice, calcium-fortified cereal products, and other calcium fortified fruit juices. If a product is fortified with calcium, it should say so on the label. Alternative sources of riboflavin, pantothenic acid, and phosphorus are found in meats, legumes (such as peanut, peas, beans, or soy), nuts, and whole grains.

Ingredient Terms You Should Know

Here is a partial list of terms commonly used on ingredient labels that indicate the presence of milk. For a milk-free diet, you should avoid foods with these ingredients:

- ➤ artificial butter flavor
- ➤ butter, butter fat, butter oil
- ➤ buttermilk
- ➤ casein
- ➤ caseinates (listed as ammonium, calcium, magnesium, potassium, or sodium caseinate)
- ➤ cheese
- ➤ cottage cheese
- ➤ cream
- ➤ curds
- ➤ custard
- ➤ ghee
- ➤ half & half
- ➤ hydrolysates (listed as casein, milk protein, protein, whey, or whey protein hydrolysate)
- ➤ lactalbumin, lactalbumin phosphate
- ➤ lactoglobulin
- ➤ lactose
- ➤ lactulose
- ➤ milk (derivative, powder, protein, solids, malted, condensed, evaporated, dry, whole, low-fat, non-fat, skimmed, and goat's milk)
- ➤ nougat

- pudding
- rennet casein
- sour cream, sour cream solids
- sour milk solids
- whey (in all forms, including sweet, delactosed, and protein concentrate)
- yogurt

The following terms *may* indicate the presence of milk:
- flavorings, including: caramel, bavarian cream, coconut cream, brown sugar, butter, and natural flavorings
- chocolate
- luncheon meat, hot dogs, sausages
- high protein flour
- margarine
- Simplesse

© The Food Allergy Network. Used with permission.

Special Concerns

Foods that may be made with milk or milk products include many baked products, such as cakes, cookies, doughnuts, and breads, frozen desserts, creamed foods, and soups. Always check the listing of ingredients carefully.

Be aware that "nondairy" products are not necessarily milk-free. Casein is a major milk allergen, and will cause a reaction in most people with a milk allergy. Unfortunately, food labeling laws consider casein or caseinates as additives even though they are milk derivatives. As a result, foods that contain these ingredients can legally be called "nondairy." Examples of nondairy foods that contain milk include: coffee whiteners, whipped toppings, imitation cheeses, soft-serve ice cream, and frozen desserts. Another concern is Asian beverages. They are made from exotic fruits which are sometimes combined with milk to make them richer.

Symbols You Should Know if You Have a Milk Allergy

Products that meet the standards of kosher dietary laws are specially marked by a rabbinical agency. Sometimes the word "kosher" is used and sometimes the agency's symbol is placed on the front of the package, usually near the product name.

The following are a few of the letters that can be found on the front of packages next to a kosher symbol and provide important information about the food's ingredients from an allergy point of view.

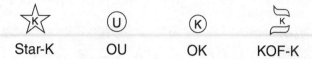

Star-K   OU   OK   KOF-K

➤ "D" indicates that a product contains dairy. These products are not safe if you have a milk allergy. Some products that list a "D" on the front and may not list milk on the ingredient statement include: tuna fish, sliced bread and bread sticks, breakfast cereals, cookies, imitation butter flavor, pancake syrup, pretzels, fruit snacks, cake mixes, and frostings.

➤ "D.E." for dairy equipment, indicates the food has been produced on equipment used to manufacture dairy-containing food. These foods are not safe for people with milk allergies.

Errors in food packaging and labeling can and do occur. Therefore, read the ingredient statement to confirm the kosher marking on the label. Bring discrepancies to the attention of the company.

Egg Allergy

If an allergy to egg white or egg yolk has been diagnosed, eggs must be avoided completely. It is impossible to separate the egg white and yolk without having some cross contamination between the two parts of the egg. This small amount of egg white or egg yolk may be enough to cause an allergic reaction.

You can replace eggs in baked goods by purchasing egg replacer, such as Jolly Joan by Ener-G Foods, or making your own. If you decide to purchase egg replacer, be sure to read the ingredient statement to be sure the product does not contain eggs. Some egg substitutes are designed for cholesterol-free diets and contain egg whites.

Eggs are not an essential food in the diet, but they do provide vitamin B_{12}, pantothenic acid, folacin, riboflavin, selenium, and biotin. Typically, these nutrients can easily be supplied by other foods in the diet, including meat and poultry products, legumes, and whole grains.

An unexpected problem which may occur with an egg-restricted diet is that your intake of grain products may be limited because many commercially prepared grain products, such as breads and pastas, contain eggs. A diet which is limited in eggs and grains may be low in some of the B vitamins and possibly iron. Read the ingredient label to find pastas and grain products made without eggs. You can also substitute rice in some recipes that call for pasta and make your own homemade bread products.

Ingredient Terms You Should Know

The following is a partial list of ingredient terms that indicate the presence of eggs and should be avoided on an egg-free diet.

- ➤ albumin
- ➤ egg (white, yolk, dried, powdered, solids)
- ➤ egg substitutes
- ➤ eggnog
- ➤ globulin
- ➤ livetin
- ➤ lysozyme (used in Europe)
- ➤ mayonnaise
- ➤ meringue
- ➤ ovalbumin
- ➤ ovomucin
- ➤ ovomucoid
- ➤ ovovitellin
- ➤ Simplesse

© The Food Allergy Network. Used with permission.

Special Concerns

Eggs are used in a wide variety of products because of their versatility. They may be used to form the custard base of ice creams and yogurts. Egg whites may be used to give pretzels, bagels, and other baked goods a shiny outer finish. Eggs are also used in coating batters for fried foods. Egg whites and shells may be used as clarifying agents in soup stocks, consumes, bouillons, and coffees. Eggs may also be found in marshmallows, marzipan, and some candies. Always be sure to read the labels.

Easy-to-Make Egg Substitutes

The following are easy-to-make egg substitutes you can use in baked goods, such as muffins, cakes, and cookies. For each egg required in a recipe, substitute one of the following:

1. 1 1/2 tablespoons water, plus 1 1/2 tablespoons oil, plus 1 teaspoon baking powder.

2. 1 teaspoon baking powder, plus 1 tablespoon water, plus 1 tablespoon vinegar.

3. 1 teaspoon yeast dissolved in 1/4 cup warm water.

4. Mix 1 packet of unflavored gelatin with 1 cup of boiling water. Substitute 3 tablespoons of this liquid for each egg. Refrigerate remainder for up to one week, and microwave to liquefy for re-use. Use in recipes with another source of leavening (i.e., baking powder or baking soda) since the gelatin functions as a binder, not a leavening agent.

© The Food Allergy Network. Used with permission.

Peanut Allergy

Peanut allergy is common in both children and adults. Peanuts are actually a legume and grow in the ground. Allergic reactions to more than one member of the legume family are rare. Other foods included in the legume family are peas, green beans, dried beans, chickpeas, and lentils. Additionally, an allergy to peanuts does not automatically mean you are allergic to tree nuts such as pecans, walnuts, or almonds.

Peanuts provide niacin, magnesium, vitamin E, manganese, and chromium. A varied diet which includes meat, whole grains, legumes, and vegetable oils can provide these same nutrients, so a peanut allergy should not result in any nutrient shortcomings.

Ingredient Terms You Should Know

The list below reveals some commonly used terms that you will find on food labels when peanut is one of the ingredients. Be sure to avoid foods with these ingredients:

➤ beer nuts
➤ cold pressed peanut oil
➤ ground nuts
➤ mixed nuts
➤ Nu-Nuts flavored nuts
➤ peanut
➤ peanut butter
➤ peanut flour

© The Food Allergy Network. Used with permission.

Special Concerns

Other places where peanuts may be found include: African, Chinese, and Thai dishes, baked goods (pastries, cookies, etc.), candy, chili, chocolate (candies, candy bars), egg rolls, hydrolyzed plant protein, hydrolyzed vegetable protein, marzipan, and nougat. Beware of artificial nuts; they can be peanuts that have been deflavored and reflavored with another nut, such as pecan or walnut.

Soybean Allergy

A soybean allergy is rare in adults. It is, however, common in infants and young children. Like peanuts, soybeans are legumes. Allergy to more than one legume is rare. In fact, many children who are allergic to soybean can eat peanuts and vice versa. As children get older, a soybean allergy is much less common than peanut allergy. Avoidance of soy is difficult because it is used in so many processed foods. For example, soybeans and soybean products are found in baked goods, canned tuna, cereals, crackers, soups, and sauces. Soy oil and soy lecithin are usually not restricted because the protein (which causes the allergy) is removed in the processing of these products.

Soybeans contribute the following nutrients: thiamin, riboflavin, vitamin B_6, folacin, calcium, phosphorus, magnesium, iron, and zinc. Even though soybeans are a nutrient-rich food, the amount of soy used in commercial products is quite small.

Thus, eliminating soy from your diet should not compromise the nutritional quality of your diet.

Ingredient Terms You Should Know

The following is a partial list of ingredient terms that indicate the presence of soy:

➤ hydrolyzed soy protein
➤ miso
➤ shoyu sauce
➤ soy (listed as soy albumin, flour, grits, nuts, milk, or sprouts)
➤ soy protein (concentrate, isolate)
➤ soy sauce
➤ soybean (granules, curd)
➤ Tamari
➤ tempeh
➤ textured vegetable protein (TVP)
➤ tofu

© The Food Allergy Network. Used with permission.

Special Concerns

Additional ingredients that may indicate the presence of soy protein in a product include: hydrolyzed plant protein, hydrolyzed vegetable protein, natural flavoring, vegetable broth, vegetable gum, vegetable starch, and flavorings.

Tree Nut Allergy

An allergy to tree nuts is one of the most common food allergies in adults. A variety of nuts have been associated with severe anaphylactic reactions. They include: almonds, Brazil nuts, cashews, chestnuts, filberts (hazelnuts), hickory nuts, macadamia nuts, pecans, pine nuts (piñon), pistachios, and walnuts.

If you have been diagnosed with an allergy to one tree nut, speak with your doctor about allergy testing to determine if you are allergic to other tree nuts.

Ingredient Terms You Should Know

Tree nuts are being added to an increasing variety of foods, making avoidance of tree nuts more difficult. The following list details some of the foods and ingredients to avoid if you have an allergy to tree nuts:

- almonds
- Brazil nuts
- cashews
- chestnuts
- filbert/hazelnuts
- gianduja (a creamy mixture of chocolate and chopped toasted nuts found in premium or imported chocolate)
- hickory nuts
- macadamia nuts
- marzipan/almond paste
- Mashuga nuts
- nougat
- Nu-Nuts artificial nuts
- nut butters (such as cashew butter)
- nut meal
- nut oil
- nut paste (such as almond paste)
- pecans (Mashuga nuts)
- pine nuts (piñon, Indian nuts, pignoli)
- pistachios
- walnuts

© The Food Allergy Network. Used with permission.

Special Concerns

Tree nuts are used in many foods, including barbecue sauce, cereals, crackers, and ice cream. Artificial nuts can be peanuts that have been deflavored and reflavored with another nut, like pecan or walnut. Pure almond extract may contain almond protein, which may cause an allergic reaction if you are allergic to almonds.

Fish Allergy

It is generally recommended that anyone who is diagnosed with a fish allergy avoid all species of fish, since the allergen is similar in the various species of fish.

Fish is a good source of protein in addition to providing niacin, vitamin B_6, vitamin B_{12}, vitamin E, phosphorus, and selenium. These nutrients are also found in meats, grains, legumes (such as peas and soybean), and oils. Therefore, it should not be too difficult to replace the nutrients found in fish.

Special Concerns

Foods which contain fish or fish products are Worcestershire sauce (if it contains anchovy), Caesar salad, caviar, and roe (fish eggs). Surimi is made from fish muscle that is reshaped and used to make imitation seafood (Alaskan pollack, a species closely related to cod, is usually used; although almost any species of fish can be used). Surimi is commonly found in imitation crab legs, lump crab meat, crab cakes, imitation lobster products, and imitation scallops. If you are allergic to fish, beware of surimi.

Shellfish Allergy

Allergic reactions to various shellfish, such as shrimp, crabs, lobster, and crawfish, and mollusks, such as clams, oysters, and scallops, are common in adults. If you have been diagnosed with an allergy to one shellfish, such as lobster, you may be allergic to other foods in the same family, such as shrimp and crab. Speak to your doctor about allergy tests to determine if you are allergic to other shellfish.

Kosher products do not contain pork or shellfish. Although imitation seafood products often contain shellfish flavors, the kosher variety is made with synthetic flavors only. Therefore, products labeled kosher should be safe for people with shellfish allergy. See page 34 for kosher symbols.

Special Concerns

Shellfish are generally not hidden in foods, however, they can be included in Asian dishes and in stuffings and not noted in the menu description of the item. Be aware that imitation seafood may not be safe for people with shellfish allergies because the flavoring used in the imitation seafood may be made from shell-fish.

Wheat Allergy

In this country, wheat is a major part of our diet, making it one of the most difficult foods to eliminate from the diet. It can be found in a wide variety of foods such as breads, cereals, pastas, crackers, snacks, lunch meats, sauces, cakes, and cookies.

Wheat is a significant source of thiamin, riboflavin, niacin, iron, selenium, and chromium. Some of these nutrients can be found in other grains that have been enriched. Enriched or fortified grain products typically include niacin, riboflavin, thiamin, and iron. Wheat is a source of several important nutrients, thus it may be useful to have a registered dietitian evaluate your diet to be sure you are getting appropriate amounts of these nutrients.

Alternative substitutes for wheat can include products made from oats, rice, rye, barley, corn, buckwheat, amaranth, and quinoa. These grains and food prepared with these grains are typically found in health food stores or via mail order specialty food companies. See the Resource Guide (Appendix 5) for the names of some specialty food companies.

Ingredient Terms You Should Know

The following is a partial listing of foods and ingredient terms that indicate the presence of wheat.

➤ bran
➤ bread crumbs
➤ bulgur
➤ cereal extract
➤ couscous
➤ cracker meal
➤ durum, durum flour
➤ enriched flour
➤ farina
➤ gluten
➤ graham flour
➤ high gluten flour
➤ high protein flour

- ➤ seitan
- ➤ semolina
- ➤ soft wheat flour
- ➤ spelt
- ➤ vital gluten
- ➤ wheat (bran, germ, gluten, malt, starch)
- ➤ whole wheat berries
- ➤ whole wheat flour

Other ingredients that *may* contain wheat protein include:
- ➤ gelatinized starch
- ➤ hydrolyzed vegetable protein
- ➤ modified food starch
- ➤ modified starch
- ➤ natural flavoring
- ➤ soy sauce
- ➤ starch
- ➤ vegetable gum
- ➤ vegetable starch

© The Food Allergy Network. Used with permission.

Special Concerns

Kamut, an ancient wheat grain, is advertised as less allergenic than wheat. However, if you are allergic to wheat, ask your doctor if you should avoid this grain. Spelt flour is also considered an ancient wheat grain. Some wheat-allergic people have reacted to this grain. If you are on a wheat-restricted diet, avoid eating spelt.

Wheat Flour Substitutes

Try substituting 1 cup of wheat flour with any one of the three recipes listed below. Experiment with a blend of flours until you get the combination you like best.

1. 1 1/3 cups rice flour

2. 1 cup barley flour

3. 3/4 cup amaranth flour plus 1/4 cup either arrowroot, tapioca, or potato starch

Less Common Causes of Food Allergy

Some of the less frequently reported food allergies include rice, corn, mustard, sesame seeds, and tropical fruits (including banana, kiwi, and mango). The following information is provided for rice and corn allergies since these are two common foods in the diet.

Rice Allergy In the United States an allergy to rice is not very common. In fact, it is the most common food offered to an infant and is often included in bland diets. However, rice allergy does exist. Rice is a source of thiamin, riboflavin, niacin, and iron, primarily via enrichment. These nutrients can also be found in enriched breads and cereals.

Ingredients that indicate the presence of rice protein are rice flour, rice starch, rice syrup, rice noodles, and rice bran.

Corn Allergy Corn allergy is rare and very difficult to manage because corn and corn products are ingredients in many food products, primarily as corn sweeteners and cornstarch. A corn-restricted diet eliminates a large variety of commercially prepared foods, including baked goods, beverages, candy, canned fruits, cereals, cookies, jams, jellies, lunch meats, snack foods, syrups, baking powder, and powdered sugar.

If you are on a corn-restricted diet, you must rely on alternative sweeteners, thickeners, and leavening agents, such as fruit juices, beet or cane sugar, maple syrup, honey, aspartame, wheat starch, potato starch, rice starch, tapioca, baking soda, and cream of tartar.

You will also find that it is necessary to make most of your own foods from scratch and not rely on commercially prepared foods. However, you may find some corn-free products in health food stores and from specialty food mail order companies.

Nutrient limitations of a corn-restricted diet are primarily due to the limited choices of food products and not by the exclusion of corn alone. Corn products contribute thiamin, riboflavin, niacin, and iron (via enrichment), and chromium to the diet. These nutrients are found in similar amounts in other enriched grain products such as hot cereals. A corn-restricted diet can potentially eliminate many foods, so a registered dietitian should evaluate your diet to be sure it is nutritionally balanced.

Chapter Five

Day-to-Day
Strategies

YOUR GOAL IN DEALING WITH FOOD ALLERGIES is to prevent a reaction. Because you encounter food in many places and situations, you'll want to have day-to-day strategies for successfully managing your food allergies. This includes how to avoid cross contamination between allergy-containing and allergy-free foods and tips for handling special occasions, traveling, and eating out. An essential part of your day-to-day strategy for coping with food allergies is to have an emergency plan of action in case you have a food allergy reaction.

Potential Sources of Cross Contamination

When a food comes into contact with another food, trace amounts, often invisible to us, of each food mix with the other. This is called cross contact or cross contamination. For people with severe food allergies, even these trace amounts can cause allergic reactions.

Cross Contamination During Processing

It is common industry practice to produce various food products on shared equipment. Government regulations require a thorough clean-up between the production of each product. However, there is a possibility that small pieces of ingredients can become lodged in the equipment during clean-up and be released during the production of the next product. In this scenario, the new product would include some ingredients which are not noted on the ingredient statement. This possibility, while rare, can pose a risk to highly allergic individuals.

Although rare, processing errors sometimes occur. If you purchase a food and find that it contains ingredients not listed on the label, save the package and call the manufacturer to report the error. After confirming the information, the company may conduct a recall of that product to prevent others from the potential of an allergic reaction.

Most adults who have a severe allergy to foods such as tree nuts and peanuts prefer to err on the side of caution and completely avoid certain types of foods. Below are examples of foods that may pose a high risk for cross contact and what causes those risks.

Candy bars, baking pieces, chocolate bars, and other candies. Plain varieties of candies and baking pieces are often run on the same line as the milk-, nut-, or peanut-containing varieties. There is a possibility that the plain items may become cross contaminated with the other varieties.

Mixed products. Most nut manufacturers process products containing peanuts and other varieties of nuts on the same production line. Food products that contain multiple ingredients, such as granola bars, can sometimes contain a stray ingredient from another product. For example, peanuts that are not listed on the ingredient list have appeared in granola bars.

Nut butters. Various types of nut butter are commonly run on shared production lines. Even though thorough cleaning is required between production of each product, there is a high chance for cross contamination from the previous product. If you have an allergy to peanuts or tree nuts, it is best to avoid these products, if possible.

Cross Contamination at Home

There are several situations which can lead to cross contact or contamination at home. Be on the lookout for these and similar instances in order to prevent a reaction.

While cooking. It is easy to accidentally use the same utensil between "safe" and "unsafe" foods during your busy time in the kitchen. As a precaution, when cooking allergy-free and allergy-containing food, cook the allergy-free meal first, cover it, and remove it from the cooking area before cooking the rest of the meal.

Re-used cooking oil. When a food, for example fish, is fried in oil, it releases some of its protein (the part of the food that causes the allergic reaction). When another food, for example French fries, is cooked in the same oil, it picks up the fish protein. As a result, anyone who is allergic to fish may have a reaction to those French fries.

During meal preparation. A knife inserted into the peanut butter jar and then used in the jelly jar will contaminate the jelly with peanut protein. That jelly may cause an allergic reaction to anyone with a peanut allergy.

Food Storage Tip

When storing foods at home, designate a special shelf in the pantry and in the refrigerator for "safe" foods. Be sure that family members all know that the food in that spot is allergy-free. Place colored stickers on food packages to mark allergy-free foods. These stickers can help children safely make their own food selections.

Cross Contamination at the Grocery Store

As you know, reading ingredient listings on food products before you buy them is an important part of managing your food allergies. Even at the grocery store, you have to use caution to avoid cross contamination between the allergy-free and allergy-containing foods you select.

Bulk food bins. Bulk food bins rarely list the ingredients of the foods, so you should avoid these foods. These bins are also a big risk for cross contamination from the other foods because you can't be sure they were thoroughly cleaned between use.

Deli meats. Cheese or milk-containing deli meats (casein, a milk protein, is often used as a binder in ham, for example) are often sliced on the same equipment as the other deli meats. As a result, the possibility of an allergic reaction from cross contamination is increased. You can avoid this risk by cooking and slicing your own deli meats. For example, bake a turkey breast, roast beef, or

Day-to-Day Strategies

chicken breast and slice it to desired thickness.

Leaking foods. The juice from allergy-free and allergy-causing foods can leak onto each other in the grocery cart. To avoid this risk secure such foods in plastic bags before placing them in the cart.

Doughnuts, muffins, and other baked goods. Different types of doughnuts, croissants, and muffins are often placed near each other in the display case. This practice makes it easy for pieces of nut toppings or milk-containing frosting to cross contaminate other foods in the display case. Additionally, if the same utensil or tissue is used to pick up the products, this also creates cross contamination possibilities.

Cross Contamination at Restaurants and Food Shops

Chinese food. Chinese foods pose a high risk if you have an allergy to nuts, fish, shellfish, or peanuts because so many of these ingredients are used in a variety of the dishes. Additionally, meals are often prepared using shared equipment and utensils. Thai and Indian foods are also high-risk foods, for the same reason. If you like this type of cookery, try cooking it at home to eliminate the risk of an allergic reaction.

Ice cream shops. Nuts and other toppings can accidentally be dropped into adjoining containers of toppings in ice cream shops. Avoid these toppings to be on the safe side.

Muffins. Store bought muffins often contain chopped or ground nuts, added for flavor and texture. Make your own muffins to be safe.

Frying oil. Most commercial cooking oils, such as soybean oil, are safe for allergic individuals because they are processed using a high heat method that removes the protein which causes the allergic reaction. However, oil that is used to fry several different foods, a common practice in restaurants, will contain protein from all those foods. As a result, if peanut-containing foods are fried in that oil, other foods will also contain peanut protein. Additionally, coldpressed, extruded, or expelled oils contain protein and may cause an allergic reaction. Most products made with cold-pressed oil indicate it on the label as an added value to that product since these oils are more expensive to use. You'll need to ask about the type of oil and frying practices before ordering food from restaurants. A safer strategy may be to avoid fried foods when eating away from home.

Candy machines. Often candy machines that contain loose candy are refilled with different products. As a result, protein residual from the old candy may contaminate the new candy.

Calling Food Manufacturers

Occasionally food labels list ingredients that may seem confusing or unclear. Do not purchase a product unless you can be absolutely sure of what all the ingredients mean. Most food products list the phone number of the manufacturers. Call them if you have any questions about their products. When calling, ask specific questions rather than general ones. Ask, "Does this product contain _____?" rather than, "What does this product contain?"

Food Labeling Regulations

The Food and Drug Administration (FDA) sets the policies for labeling requirements for packaged foods. Currently, the FDA requires that manufacturers list all ingredients present in products. However, according to the "Two Percent Rule," ingredients present in small amounts, 2 percent or less of weight, do not have to be listed in rank order. In these cases, the listing of these ingredients is placed at the end of the ingredient statement following a quantifying statement, such as, "contains ___ percent or less of _____."

There are some exceptions to this rule, however. One exception applies to incidental additives. Incidental additives do not have to be declared at all if they are not functional in the finished product and are present in insignificant amounts. "Insignificant" is not defined, but industry practice seems to be in the parts per million range.

Additionally, ingredients used in the "flavors" or "spices" listed on food labels are not required to be listed separately. This practice protects the secret recipes that make each company's product unique. Furthermore, most manufacturers buy flavors and spices from companies that specialize in making these recipes.

The flavor houses also consider each recipe their own secret. Unfortunately, flavors can include such foods as peanuts or milk. For some allergic individuals even these small amounts can cause a reaction. As manufacturers and flavor houses become more aware of food allergies and the potential seriousness of reactions, many are voluntarily listing ingredients on the label even when they are present in very small amounts.

Food Manufacturer Initiatives

Most of the large manufacturers are conducting in-depth reviews of their production schedules and labeling policies from a food allergy perspective. They are attempting to limit the production of foods containing the major allergens to either specific production lines or times. This will reduce the risk of cross contamination of their products.

In addition they are changing their labeling policies to clearly declare allergen containing ingredients not only on the ingredient list but on other areas of the package, such as below the ingredient listing with the statement "contains _____ ingredients." Foods that are produced on the same lines as allergen-containing foods may be labeled as "may contain _____." These new practices should help you easily spot offending foods on ingredient statements.

Manufacturers are also developing training materials for their employees in order to educate them about food allergies and the important role employees play in providing safe foods for the consumer.

Traveling and Eating Out

Equally as important as managing day-to-day activities is a plan for handling special occasions, such as travel and eating away from home. Use these strategies and tips to help ensure that you enjoy your special occasions.

Traveling Tips

➤ Make a list of points needing close attention well in advance of traveling. Keep a list and check it before you leave to be sure you haven't forgotten anything.
➤ Be sure the people traveling with you know the symptoms you may have during an allergic reaction. Teach them what

to do if you have a reaction. See the Emergency Plan (page 53) for guidelines.

➤ Discuss your travel plans with your doctor. Be sure you have necessary medications and updated prescriptions.

➤ If you are traveling by public transportation and have to check your luggage, keep any prescribed medications, such as EpiPen or Ana Guard, with you.

➤ Keep some "safe" food with you just in case you are delayed in reaching your destination. Having your own food allows you to retain control of what you eat and minimizes the stress of seeking out an eatery that has food you can safely eat.

➤ Try to avoid staying with people who don't understand your diet restrictions. It is best to visit them before or after mealtime, so you won't have to worry about a potential reaction.

Eating Out Tips

➤ Because restaurants are often very busy on Fridays, Saturdays, and Sundays, your special meal request will more likely be welcomed and delivered accurately on a less popular day, such as Monday.

➤ Before eating at a new restaurant, review the menu to be sure there is something you can eat. Keep in mind that the same dish in two different restaurants may have different ingredients. Always ask questions.

➤ Ask about ingredients and preparation methods before you order. Although food preparation in fast food restaurant chains is usually standardized, there can be regional differences across the country.

➤ When choosing a restaurant in your hometown, the best place to go is one where you are known so that you can be sure your special meal request will be honored. If there is a restaurant in your area that you and your family enjoy, get to know the manager or owner and let them know your special needs.

Recipe Surprises

Chefs are hired because of their creativity. However, sometimes their creative use of a common food can create a problem for unsuspecting consumers with food allergies. Below are examples of recipe surprises—unusual ways that potential allergens may be used—reported from some restaurants. Be sure to ask about ingredients as you order food in restaurants. You'll probably come across many more recipe surprises.

➤ Peanut butter has been combined with cocoa mix and hot water to add extra flavor.

➤ Peanut butter can be an ingredient in a sauce or marinade recipe on skewered turkey or chicken pieces.

➤ Peanut flour has been used as the special thickener in sauce for ribs.

➤ Pine nuts have been used in strawberry sauce to improve the flavor. Pine nuts are also being used more frequently in salad dressing and spaghetti sauces.

➤ Many steak restaurants put butter on top of steaks right after they've been grilled. The butter adds extra flavor and makes a well-cooked steak more juicy. After the butter melts, it is not visible.

➤ Asian cookery may offer some meatless versions of old favorites, such as a spicy "beef" fried with lemon grass. Beware—these dishes are often made with wheat. The flour is sometimes flavored and shaped to look like beef, pork, and shrimp.

➤ Some local bakery stores add wheat to their rye bread. When shopping at small stores or specialty shops, or when buying products that are not packaged with an ingredient list, always ask about ingredients used.

➤ Soybeans can be shaped to look like chicken for some Asian dishes.

➤ Soy protein and soy flours are being used more often in baked goods. An example is soy-containing pizza dough used in Mexican pizza.

➤ Eggs are sometimes used to hold meatballs together. They are also used to add a golden glaze to baked goods.

An Emergency Plan

Despite your best efforts to avoid eating a food to which you are allergic, accidents can occur. If a reaction occurs, quick action is key in order to avoid discomfort and a potentially life-threatening medical emergency. You'll need to develop an emergency plan of action.

An effective emergency plan should include the following basic information:

1. A list of foods to which you are allergic.
2. A list of prescribed medications and the dose needed if you have a reaction.
3. The usual symptoms you might have if you are having an allergic reaction.
4. A step-by-step plan of what should be done to treat the reaction, including the sequence of medications that should be given.
5. The names and phone numbers of three emergency contacts in case you are unable to speak. (Having more than one person on your list makes it more likely that someone will be reached when you need it.)
6. The name and phone number of your doctor and the closest emergency medical care facility to your home.
7. A written statement from your doctor outlining how the doctor wants your reaction to be treated. For example, if you commonly have mild symptoms at first that quickly get worse, the doctor may not want others to "wait and see." This step is particularly important if you have severe reactions, if you travel frequently, and are likely to be out of reach of your doctor. Having a written statement will prevent you from having to convince another health care professional that you know what you need.

Keep your emergency plan of action with your antihistamine or epinephrine kit, EpiPen or Ana Guard, if the doctor has prescribed them. And always carry the emergency plan and your medications with you.

An EpiPen trainer, without medication and a needle, is available so that you and others close to you can become comfortable with giving this type of injection. Contact the Food Allergy

Network (see Appendix 5) for a trainer if your doctor does not have one available for you. Finally, check expiration dates regularly because expired medication may not treat the reaction effectively.

If the allergic person is a child, be sure to provide the emergency information to various people who regularly care for your child, such as school personnel (principal, teachers, nurses), babysitters, neighbors, friends, and relatives. If your child has severe allergies, medications should always go where the child goes, even if you don't expect food to be served. It doesn't hurt to be very cautious.

A Medic Alert bracelet or necklace will also help identify your special needs in case of a medical emergency. The jewelry can be ordered directly from the company. See the Resource Guide for details.

Remember, it's best to be prepared and not need to use your emergency plan than to have a reaction and not know what to do.

How to Keep
a Diet Diary

TO EVALUATE POSSIBLE REACTIONS TO FOODS, you may be asked to keep a diet diary. This will involve keeping a record of what you eat for several days, usually 3 or 7 days. Here are instructions and a sample diet diary form for a 3-day diet diary:

1. Record everything you eat and drink for three consecutive days, even if it's a small bite of a food. Try to keep your record for two weekdays and one weekend day (for example, Thursday, Friday, and Saturday or Sunday, Monday, and Tuesday). Do not record on holidays, vacation, or sick days.

2. Record the information in the appropriate column. Be specific about brand names and methods of preparation. See sample on page 56.

3. Measure amounts or estimate portion sizes in common measurements (for example, fluid ounces, ounces, cups, teaspoons, etc.).

4. Remember to include all condiments, such as sugar, jelly, margarine, mayonnaise, catsup, dressings, sauces, etc.

5. Be sure to accurately record the time the food was eaten.

6. Record any vitamin/mineral supplements taken in measured amounts or as number of pills/capsules. Also include brand name.

Name
Date

Sample

Meal or Snack and Time Eaten	Food or Drink Served	Brand Name/ How Prepared	Condiments Added	Amount Eaten	Symptoms Noted
BREAKFAST 7:30 AM	1 cup orange juice	Minute Maid concentrate, diluted per directions		1/2 cup	
8:30 AM	1 cup Rice Krispies	Kellogg's		all	
	1/2 cup whole milk	store brand		1/4 cup	
	1 slice white toast	store brand	1 tsp butter	all	
	6-inch banana	peeled		all	Cheeks became red, stomach pains and nausea
SNACK 10:00 AM	1 apple, (2 1/2" diam.)	raw, peeled		1/2	
	1 Tbsp. peanut butter	Peter Pan, reduced fat		all	
10:30 AM	1 cup apple juice	Motts, canned		3/4 cup	vomited all the snack

Food Allergies

56

Day 1

Name _____
Date _____

Meal or Snack and Time Eaten	Food or Drink Served	Brand Name/ How Prepared	Condiments Added	Amount Eaten	Symptoms Noted
BREAKFAST					
SNACK					

How to Keep a Diet Diary

Day 1

Name _____

Date _____

Meal or Snack and Time Eaten	Food or Drink Served	Brand Name/ How Prepared	Condiments Added	Amount Eaten	Symptoms Noted
LUNCH					
SNACK					

Name _____
Date _____

Meal or Snack and Time Eaten	Food or Drink Served	Brand Name/ How Prepared	Condiments Added	Amount Eaten	Symptoms Noted
DINNER					
SNACK					

Day 1

Vitamins, Minerals, and Other Supplements

Time	Amount Taken

How to Keep a Diet Diary

Name _____

Date _____

Day 2

Meal or Snack and Time Eaten	Food or Drink Served	Brand Name/ How Prepared	Condiments Added	Amount Eaten	Symptoms Noted
BREAKFAST					
SNACK					

Name _____

Date _____

Day 2

Meal or Snack and Time Eaten	Food or Drink Served	Brand Name/ How Prepared	Condiments Added	Amount Eaten	Symptoms Noted
LUNCH					
SNACK					

Name _____

Date _____

Day 2

Meal or Snack and Time Eaten	Food or Drink Served	Brand Name/ How Prepared	Condiments Added	Amount Eaten	Symptoms Noted
DINNER					
SNACK					

Vitamins, Minerals, and Other Supplements	Time	Amount Taken

Food Allergies

62

Name _____

Date _____

Day 3

Meal or Snack and Time Eaten	Food or Drink Served	Brand Name/ How Prepared	Condiments Added	Amount Eaten	Symptoms Noted
BREAKFAST					
SNACK					

How to Keep a Diet Diary

Name _____

Date _____

Day 3

Meal or Snack and Time Eaten	Food or Drink Served	Brand Name/ How Prepared	Condiments Added	Amount Eaten	Symptoms Noted
LUNCH					
SNACK					

Food Allergies

64

Name

Date

Day 3

Meal or Snack and Time Eaten	Food or Drink Served	Brand Name/ How Prepared	Condiments Added	Amount Eaten	Symptoms Noted
DINNER					
SNACK					

Vitamins, Minerals, and Other Supplements

Time

Amount Taken

How to Keep a Diet Diary

Appendix Two

Sample Menus

THIS SERIES OF MENUS was developed as a trial elimination diet. Its use should be limited to a 2- to 4-week period, after which all food restrictions should be confirmed with a double blind placebo controlled food challenge (see Chapter 2). These menus provide a well balanced, nutritionally complete meal plan. All of the major food allergens (milk, egg, soy, peanut, nuts, fish, shellfish, and wheat) have been eliminated from these meal plans using homemade allergy-free recipes. These meals provide an average of 2300 calories per day. Portion sizes may be adjusted to meet your individual calorie needs.

The enriched milk substitute refers to beverages such as rice milk which have been enriched with vitamins A and D and calcium. The enrichment provides amounts of these vitamins and calcium that would be present in milk. If you are between the age of 11 and 24 years or are a nursing mother you will need to add one more cup of enriched milk substitute daily to meet your body's calcium needs.

Day 1

Breakfast
   1 cup apple juice
   3 oatmeal pancakes with 1 Tbsp. unsalted, milk- and soy-free
      margarine
   1/2 cup canned peaches

4 slices bacon
1 cup enriched milk substitute

Lunch
4 ounces sliced fresh ham
2 corn rice muffins (see p. 75)
1 ounce potato chips
1 apple
1 cup enriched milk substitute

Dinner
1 1/2 cups rice pasta with
   1 cup regular tomato sauce and
   3 ounces ground turkey
1/2 cup cooked carrots
1/2 cup cooked spinach
2 tsp. vegetable oil
1 cup enriched milk substitute

Snack
1 fresh orange

Day 2

Breakfast
1/2 cup cubed melon
1 cup cream of rice cereal with
   1 tsp. unsalted, milk- and soy-free margarine
2 oat muffins with jelly and
   2 tsp. unsalted, milk- and soy-free margarine
1 cup enriched milk substitute

Lunch
3 ounces sliced turkey breast
1 cup white rice
1/2 cup cranberry sauce
1/2 cup cooked squash
2 tsp. vegetable oil
1 cup enriched milk substitute

Dinner

4 ounces cooked sliced fresh ham
1 baked sweet potato with
  2 tsp. unsalted, milk- and soy-free margarine
1 cup enriched milk substitute
1/2 cup pineapple

Snack

1 fresh pear

Day 3

Breakfast

1 cup orange juice
1 cup puffed rice cereal with
  1 cup enriched milk substitute
1 ounce sliced grilled ham
1 banana rice muffin

Lunch

3 ounces ground lamb patty
2 slices egg-, milk-, and wheat-free bread
10 French fried potatoes
1 banana
1 cup enriched milk substitute

Dinner

3 ounces broiled pork chop
1 cup white rice with
  1 tsp. unsalted, milk- and soy-free margarine
1/2 cup steamed broccoli
1 tsp. vegetable oil
1 cup enriched milk substitute

Snack

1 fresh apple

Day 4

Breakfast
1 cup apple juice
1 cup oatmeal
1 banana
2 ounces pork sausage patties
1 cup enriched milk substitute

Lunch
3 ounces hamburger patty
2 slices egg-, milk-, and wheat-free bread
1 ounce potato chips
1/2 cup cooked peas
1 tsp. vegetable oil
1 cup enriched milk substitute

Dinner
3 ounces chicken breast
1 cup white rice with
   2 tsp. unsalted milk- and soy-free margarine
1/2 cup cooked green beans
1 small tossed green salad with
   oil and vinegar dressing
1 cup enriched milk substitute

Snack
1 fresh tangerine

Day 5

Breakfast
1/2 cup fresh fruit salad
2 potato pancakes with
   2 tsp. unsalted milk- and soy-free margarine
1 cup enriched milk substitute

Lunch
Homemade beef stew made with
   3 ounces cubed beef

1/2 cup cubed potatoes
1/2 cup diced carrots
1 fresh apple
1 cup enriched milk substitute

Dinner
3 ounces lamb chop
1/2 cup mashed potatoes
1/2 cup cooked spinach
2 tsp. vegetable oil
1/2 cup fresh pineapple
1 cup enriched milk substitute

Snack
1 fresh banana

Day 6

Breakfast
1 cup grape juice
1 cup corn grits cereal
2 tsp. unsalted, milk- and soy-free margarine
2 ounces grilled ham
1 cup enriched milk substitute

Lunch
Chicken, vegetable, and rice soup made with
   3 ounces baked chicken breast
   1/3 cup white rice
   1 cup chicken broth
   1 cup julienne mixed vegetables
   1 tsp. vegetable oil
1 corn rice muffin (see p. 75)
1 banana
1 cup enriched milk substitute

Dinner
1 cup of rice pasta with
1 cup of peppers, green beans, and carrots sautéed in 1 Tbsp.
   vegetable oil
4 ounces sirloin steak strips

1 slice milk-, egg-, and wheat-free bread
1 tsp. unsalted milk- and soy-free margarine
1/2 cup fresh fruit cocktail
1 cup enriched milk substitute

Snack
1 fresh orange

Day 7

Breakfast
1 banana
1 cup puffed corn cereal
1 apple rice muffin
2 ounces pork sausage patty
1 cup enriched milk substitute

Lunch
3 ounces grilled chicken breast
2 slices egg-, milk-, wheat-, and soy-free bread
10 French fries
1 tossed green salad with oil and vinegar dressing
1/2 cup canned pears
1 cup enriched milk substitute

Dinner
3 ounces roast pork
1/2 cup mashed sweet potatoes
1/2 cup cooked broccoli
2 tsp. vegetable oil
1/2 cup fresh fruit salad
1 cup enriched milk substitute

Snack
1/2 cup grapes

Appendix Three
Allergy-Free
Recipes

COOKING FOR A FOOD-RESTRICTED DIET can take some practice, but you'll find that once you learn appropriate substitutions for an allergy-causing food, you can easily adapt your favorite recipes to make meals the whole family will enjoy. Check your local bookstore or contact some of the resource organizations in Appendix 5 for recipes and suggested resources. Below are some simple recipes to get you started. Be sure to read ingredient labels carefully for all foods.

Key to Symbols:

M = Milk-free	P = Peanut-free
E = Egg-free	S = Soy-free
W = Wheat-free	N = Nut-free

Recipes used with permission. © *The Food Allergy News Cookbook.*

Pancakes or Waffles
M, E, P, S, N

2 cups flour
4 tsp. baking powder
1/2 tsp. salt
2 Tbsp. sugar

2 cups water
3 Tbsp. oil
1/4 tsp. vanilla extract

Sift together dry ingredients. Add remaining ingredients and beat together. Pour the batter onto a hot, lightly greased griddle or heavy skillet forming circles approximately 4 inches in diameter. Cook for 5 minutes or until pancakes have a bubbly surface and slightly dry edges. Turn pancakes; cook 2 to 3 minutes more or until golden brown. Makes 8 to 12, 4-inch pancakes or waffles.

Suggestions: For a special treat for kids, pour this batter onto a hot griddle in a teddy bear, bunny, or other fun shape. Add banana slices, blueberries, or other fruit to batter for variety.

English Muffin Bread
M, E, P, S, N

2 packages active dry yeast
6 cups unsifted flour
1/4 tsp. baking soda
1 Tbsp. sugar

2 tsp. salt
2 1/2 cups water
cornmeal

Combine yeast, 3 cups flour, baking soda, sugar, and salt. Heat water until very warm (120–130°F). Add to dry mixture; beat well. Stir in remaining flour gradually to make a stiff batter. Spoon into two 8 1/2 x 4 1/2 inch loaf pans that have been greased with an allowed oil or shortening and sprinkle with cornmeal. Sprinkle tops with cornmeal.

Cover, and let rise in a warm place for 45 minutes. Bake at 400°F for 25 minutes. Remove from pans immediately and cool. This bread toasts and freezes well.

M = Milk-free; E = Egg-free; W = Wheat-free; P = Peanut-free; S = Soy-free; N = Nut-free

Corn Rice Muffins
M, E, W, P, S, N

1/3 cup vegetable shortening
1/4 cup sugar
2/3 cup cream of rice cereal, dry
2/3 cup warm water
1 Tbsp. baking powder

1/4 tsp. salt
1 tsp. vanilla extract
1 tsp. grated lemon rind
2/3 cup cornmeal

Preheat oven to 375°F. Cream shortening and sugar. In a separate bowl, combine rice cereal, warm water, baking powder, and salt; add to sugar mixture. Mix in remaining ingredients just until dry ingredients are incorporated. Spoon into greased muffin tins (make small muffins for better texture). Bake for 25 minutes. Makes 8 muffins.

Deep Dish Pizza Dough
M, E, P, S, N

1 package dry yeast
1 cup water
1/4 cup vegetable oil
2 Tbsp. olive oil

1/4 cup cornmeal
2 3/4 cups flour, divided into
    1 3/4 cups and 1 cup

Dissolve yeast in warm water (120 to 130°F). Add oils, cornmeal, and 1 3/4 cups flour. Beat for 10 minutes with an electric mixer. Add remaining flour; knead 10 to 15 minutes. If dough is sticky, add a few tablespoons flour. Let rise in a warm place until doubled. Punch down, then let rise again until almost doubled.

Preheat oven to 475°F. Oil two 10-inch cake pans (or a 12-inch pizza pan for thin crust pizza). Divide dough in half, place in center of each pan, and press to about 1/4-inch thickness, pushing dough up on sides of the pans. Top with spaghetti sauce and other desired toppings. Bake 20 to 30 minutes for the deep dish pizzas (depending on the toppings added) and 10 to 15 minutes for a thin crust pizza.

M = Milk-free; E = Egg-free; W = Wheat-free; P = Peanut-free; S = Soy-free; N = Nut-free

Puffed Rice Treats
M, E, W, P, S, N

1/2 stick milk- and soy-free margarine
40 regular-size egg-free, milk-free marshmallows

5 cups puffed rice cereal

Grease a 13 x 9 inch pan and set aside. Melt margarine and add marshmallows. Heat and stir mixture until melted. Add puffed rice. Press into the well-greased pan. Allow to cool, then cut into squares.

Gingersnap Cookies
M, E, W, P, S, N

3/4 cup milk- and soy-free margarine
1 cup brown sugar
1/4 cup molasses
2 Tbsp. orange juice
2 1/4 cups barley flour

2 tsp. baking soda
1/2 tsp. salt
1 tsp. ground ginger
1 tsp. ground cinnamon
1/2 tsp. ground cloves
sugar

Preheat oven to 375°F. Cream together the margarine, brown sugar, molasses, and orange juice. In a separate bowl, sift together flour, baking soda, salt, ground ginger, ground cinnamon, and ground cloves. Add the dry ingredients to the molasses mixture and mix well.

Form into small balls. Roll in granulated sugar and place 2 inches apart on a greased cookie sheet. Bake 12 minutes. Makes about 5 dozen cookies.

Vanilla Frosting
M, E, W, P, S, N

2/3 cup solid vegetable shortening
1 lb. box confectioners sugar

3 Tbsp. water
1 tsp. imitation vanilla extract

Cream shortening until smooth. Add sugar, and cream mixture until well blended. Add water. Beat until smooth. Chill at least 1 hour. Beat again and add vanilla extract.

M = Milk-free; E = Egg-free; W = Wheat-free; P = Peanut-free; S = Soy-free; N = Nut-free

Oatmeal Cookies
M, E, W, P, S, N

1/2 cup brown sugar
1/2 cup granulated sugar
1/2 cup milk- and soy-free
  margarine
1 tsp. vanilla extract
1 Tbsp. water
1 1/2 Tbsp. water mixed with
  1 1/2 Tbsp. oil, and 1 tsp.
  baking powder

1 cup oat flour (oatmeal ground
  to flour consistency)
1/2 tsp. baking soda
1/2 tsp. baking powder
1/2 tsp. salt
2 cups quick oats

Preheat oven to 350°F. Grease cookie sheets with allowed short-ening or oil. Cream together sugars and margarine. Add vanilla, water, and baking powder mixture; beat until smooth. Sift together flour, baking soda, baking powder, and salt. Add to wet ingredients; mix until smooth. Add oats, and mix well. Drop by teaspoonfuls, 2 inches apart, onto greased cookie sheet. Bake 10 minutes or until lightly browned. Let cool before removing from cookie sheets. Makes about 3 dozen cookies.

Fried Ripe Bananas
M, E, W, P, S, N

1 banana
1 cup barley flour
1 cup water
1 Tbsp. sugar

1/8 tsp. cinnamon
2 Tbsp. milk- and soy-free
  margarine
1/4 cup sugar

Cut the banana into 1/4-inch slices. Set aside. In an air-tight con-tainer, mix together flour, water, sugar, and cinnamon. Add banana slices. Cover and shake gently until the bananas are well coated. Set aside. Melt margarine in a frying pan. Add the bananas and fry until browned, gently turning bananas once. Remove from pan, and roll in sugar.

Serve with hot cereal for breakfast or as a dessert.

M = Milk-free; E = Egg-free; W = Wheat-free; P = Peanut-free; S = Soy-free; N = Nut-free

George Washington's Cherry Cookies
M, E, P, S, N

1/2 cup milk- and soy-free
   margarine, softened
1/2 cup sugar
1 1/2 Tbsp. oil mixed with
   1 1/2 Tbsp. water, and 1 tsp.
   baking powder

1/2 tsp. vanilla extract
1 cup flour
1/4 cup cocoa powder
1/2 cup maraschino cherries,
   chopped

Preheat oven to 350°F. Grease cookie sheets. Blend together margarine and sugar. Stir in baking powder mixture and vanilla extract. Add flour and cocoa powder and mix thoroughly. Stir in cherries. Drop dough by teaspoonfuls 1 inch apart onto cookie sheet. Bake 15 minutes or until cookies are firm. Cool slightly and remove from baking pans. Makes approximately 2 dozen cookies.

Halloween Cookies
M, E, P, S, N

3 cups flour
1 Tbsp. pumpkin pie spice
1 Tbsp. ground ginger
1/2 tsp. salt
1 cup milk- and soy-free
   margarine

2 cups sugar
1 cup canned pumpkin
1 1/2 Tbsp. oil mixed with
   1 1/2 Tbsp. water and 1 tsp.
   baking powder

In a medium bowl, combine flour, pumpkin pie spice, ginger, and salt; set aside. In a large mixer bowl, cream margarine and sugar until fluffy. Add canned pumpkin and baking powder mixture and mix until combined. Add dry ingredients and mix well. Cover and chill in refrigerator until dough is firm.

Preheat oven to 350°F. Drop dough by rounded teaspoonfuls onto greased cookie sheets. Flatten slightly. Create a "stem" with dough and press into top of cookie. Bake 16 minutes, or until lightly browned. Makes approximately 4 dozen cookies.

Cool on wire racks. Frost in a pumpkin design using orange and green frosting.

M = Milk-free; E = Egg-free; W = Wheat-free; P = Peanut-free; S = Soy-free; N = Nut-free

Chocolate Wacky Cupcakes

M, E, W, P, S, N

2 cups rice flour
1 cup sugar
1/2 tsp. salt
3 Tbsp. unsweetened cocoa
    powder

1 tsp. baking soda
1 tsp. vanilla extract
1 Tbsp. vinegar
5 Tbsp. oil
1 cup cold water

Preheat oven to 350°F. Line muffin pans with foil liners. Set aside. In a large mixing bowl, stir together flour, sugar, salt, cocoa, and baking soda. Add vanilla extract, vinegar, oil, and water. Mix thoroughly. Pour batter into prepared pans and bake 25 to 30 minutes or until done. Makes 12 cupcakes.

Chocolate Pound Cake

M, E, P, S, N

3/4 cup milk- and soy-free
    margarine, softened
1 1/2 cups sugar
4 1/2 Tbsp. water mixed with
    4 1/2 Tbsp. oil and 3 tsp.
    baking powder
3 1/2 cups flour
3/4 cup unsweetened cocoa
    powder

1 tsp. baking powder
1/4 tsp. salt
1 1/2 cups water
1 tsp. baking soda
2 tsp. vanilla extract
1 Tbsp. confectioners' sugar

Preheat oven to 350°F. Grease a Bundt pan with an allowed oil or shortening and set aside. In a large mixing bowl, cream together margarine and sugar. Add baking powder mixture. Mix well and set aside. In a separate bowl, combine flour, cocoa, baking powder, and salt. Add dry ingredients to creamed mixture and mix well. In a medium bowl, combine water and baking soda, and add to flour and margarine mixture. Stir in vanilla extract and blend well. Pour into Bundt pan. Bake 45 minutes or until a knife or wooden pick inserted in center comes out clean. Cool in pan 10 minutes. Remove from pan and cool completely on wire rack. Top cake with confectioners' sugar.

M = Milk-free; E = Egg-free; W = Wheat-free; P = Peanut-free; S = Soy-free; N = Nut-free

Appendix Four

Glossary of Allergy Terms

BELOW ARE DEFINITIONS for words commonly used by allergists in describing their diagnosis.

Angioedema Swelling of the skin and underlying tissue.

Antibody A protein in the bloodstream or other body fluids that is produced in response to foreign materials that enter the body; antibodies usually protect us.

Antigen Any substance that causes an immune system response when introduced into the body.

Antihistamine A drug that blocks the effects of histamine, a chemical which is responsible for many of the symptoms of allergy when released by the body during an allergic reaction.

Atopic Dermatitis A chronic, itching inflammation of the skin; also referred to as eczema.

DBPCFC Acronym for double-blind, placebo-controlled food challenge. A diagnostic procedure whereby neither the doctor nor the patient knows what is being tested. This is the gold standard for food allergy testing, used to confirm the results of positive skin tests.

Histamine A chemical released by the body and considered responsible for much of the swelling and itching characteristic of hay fever and other allergies.

Prick Skin Test A skin test in which a drop of allergen is placed on the skin and then pricked with a needle. If the patient is allergic to that substance, a small raised area surrounded by redness will appear at the test site within 15 minutes.

RAST Test A blood test which can detect the presence of allergic antibody in the blood.

Rhinitis An inflammation of the membrane lining the nose. Allergic rhinitis is also called hay fever.

Scratch Test A skin test in which the skin is lightly scratched and a drop of the allergen is placed on the scratched area.

Uticaria Hives; a reaction in the skin marked by swelling, redness, and itching.

Appendix Five

Resource Guide

To find a board-certified allergist, contact:

American Academy of Allergy, Asthma & Immunology
611 East Wells Street
Milwaukee, WI 53202
(800) 822-2762
(414) 272-6071
Web Site: www.aaaai.org

American College of Asthma, Allergy and Immunology
85 West Algonquin Road, Suite 550
Arlington Heights, IL 60005
(800) 842-7777
Web Site: www.allergy.mcg.edu

To find a board-certified pediatrician, contact:

American Academy of Pediatrics
141 Northwest Point Boulevard
P.O. Box 927
Elk Grove Village, IL 60009
(800) 433-9016
Web Site: www.aap.org

To find a registered dietitian:

The American Dietetic Association
216 West Jackson Boulevard
Chicago, IL 60606-6995
(800) 366-1655
Web Site: www.eatright.org

Or (900)CALL-AN-RD (900/225-5267) for customized answers to your food and nutrition questions.

Nonprofit organizations:

Allergy and Asthma Network/Mothers of Asthmatics, Inc.
3554 Chain Bridge Road, Suite 200
Fairfax, VA 22030
(800) 878-4403
(703) 385-4403
Web Site: www.podi.com/health/aanma

Provides monthly newsletter and other educational materials for managing asthma and allergies.

Asthma and Allergy Foundation of America
1125 15th Street, NW, Suite 502
Washington, DC 20056
(800) 7-ASTHMA
(202) 466-7643
Fax: (202) 466-8940

Dedicated to finding a cure for and controlling asthma and allergic diseases. Has a network of chapters and support groups located throughout the nation.

Asthma/Allergy Information Association
30 Eglinton Avenue West, Suite 750
Mississauga, Ontario CANADA L5R 3E7
(905) 712-2242
(905) 712-2245

Provides patient education, newsletters, and other materials for managing asthma and allergies.

Celiac Sprue Association/United States of America, Inc.
P.O. Box 31700
Omaha, NE 68131-0700
(402) 558-0600

Provides information and referral services for persons with celiac sprue, including gluten-free diets, gluten-free commercial foods, and gluten-free medications.

Celiac Disease Foundation
13251 Ventura Boulevard, Suite 3
Studio City, CA 91504-1838
(818) 990-2354
(818) 990-2379

Services and support to persons with celiac disease and dermatitis herpetiformis through programs of awareness, education, advocacy, and research.

The Food Allergy Network
10400 Eaton Place, Suite 107
Fairfax, Virginia 22030-2208
(800) 929-4040
(703) 691-3179
Fax: (703) 691-2713
Web Site: www.foodallergy.org

Devoted solely to patient education for food allergy and anaphylaxis, a potentially life-threatening allergic reaction. FAN provides videos, pamphlets, cookbooks, newsletters, How to Read a Label cards, patient conferences, and EpiPen trainers. Free information is available to callers.

International Food Information Council Foundation
1100 Connecticut Avenue, NW, Suite 430
Washington, DC 20036
(202) 296-6540
(202) 296-6547
Web Site: ificinfo.health.org

Provides sound, scientific information on food safety and nutrition to journalists, health professionals, educators, government officials, and consumers.

Medic Alert Foundation United States
2323 Colorado Avenue
Turlock, CA 95382
(209) 668-3333
(209) 669-2495

Provides quick, accessible, vital personal medical information to protect its members and save lives in emergency situations from any phone around the world.

National Eczema Association
1221 SW Yamhill, #303
Portland, OR 97205
(503) 228-4430

Dedicated to atopic dermatitis education and research. Provides educational and informational services, working to increase public awareness, and support training and research.

Specialty Food Companies:

Ener-G Foods, Inc.
5960 1st Avenue, South
P.O. Box 84487
Seattle, WA 98124-5787
(206) 767-6660
Fax: (206) 764-3398
Web Site: www.ener-g.com

Manufacturer of specialty diet foods for over 75 years. Foods can be ordered via mail or purchased in large health food stores. Includes wheat-free breads, doughnuts, and cookies; egg replacer; and premixed dough for cakes and muffins. Detailed information concerning product ingredients and nutrients and a free catalog is available.

Miss Roben's
P.O. Box 1434
Frederick, MD 21702
(800) 891-0083
Fax: (301) 631-5954
E-mail: missroben@msn.com

Specializes in wheat-free bread, cake, and cookie mixes. Ready-to-eat gluten- and wheat-free foods such as pizzas, pasta, muffins, and other baking items also available. Custom mixes are also available upon special request.

The Gluten-Free Pantry
P.O. Box 840
Glastonbury, CT 06033
(800) 291-8386
Web Site: www.glutenfree.com

Specializes in bread and pizza mixes. Specialty flours, such as rice, tapioca, and potato flour; baking pans, and cookbooks also available. Provides recipes for cooking without wheat or gluten. Catalog available.

Additional References:

Bock, M.D., S. Allan, *Food Allergy: A Primer for People*, Vantage Press, Inc., 1988.

Muñoz-Furlong, A., Goldberg, E., *Students With Food Allergies: What Do the Laws Say?*, The Food Allergy Network, 1994.

Muñoz-Furlong, A., *The School Food Allergy Program*, The Food Allergy Network, 1995.

Index

minerals, children and, 28

Miss Roben's, 87

myths, food allergy, ix

National Eczema Association, 86

nausea, 2

Neocate, 21

Nutramigen, 21

nutrient requirements, children and, 26–28

nutritional status, children's, 22–23, 24–26

nuts, 3, 38–39, 52

open challenge test, 12

oral allergy syndrome, 7

pain, abdominal, 2

peanut allergy, 3, 21, 36–37, 52
  contamination risks and, 46
  ingredients to avoid, 37
  prevalence of, 2

pediatrician, finding a, 83

penicillin, 3

Pregestimil, 21

preservatives, ix

prevalence rates, food allergies, ix, 2, 4

prick skin test, 11–12
  definition of, 82

protein, children and, 27

protocolitis, food-induced, 5

radioallergosorbent test (RAST), 11
  definition of, 82

ragweed allergy, 7

rash, 1

RAST (radioallergosorbent test), 11
  definition of, 82

reactions, allergic
  avoiding contaminants, 45–49
  biphasic, 15
  causes of, 1
  children and, 54
  digestive tract, 2
  emergency preparations and, 53–54
  false positive, 11
  life-threatening, 3
  onset of, 2
  respiratory tract, 2
  signs in children, 23–24
  skin, 1, 81, 82
  treatment methods, 14, 17

recipes, allergy-free, 73–79

recordkeeping, 17, 25–26, 55–65

resources, 83–87

respiratory tract reactions, 2

restaurant dining, 48–49, 50–52

rhinitis, 82

rice allergy, 43

scratch test, 82

serum IgE concentration, 10

shellfish allergy, 3–4, 40–41

shock, anaphylactic, 3

shopping, grocery, avoiding contaminants and, 47–48

shrimp, 4

skin reactions, 1, 81, 82
  treating, 14–15

soybean allergy, 3, 37–38, 52
  ingredients to avoid, 38

spices, ix

steroids, 15

subcutaneous testing, 14

sublingual testing, 13

sulfite-induced asthma, 5

sulfite-sensitivity, 6

sulfites, 5–6

surimi, 40

swelling, mouth and facial, 1

symptoms, allergic, 2–3, 14–15.
See also reactions

tests, allergy, 9–14, 82
    unproven, 13–14

throat problems, 2

travel, strategies for, 50–51

tree nut allergy, 3, 21, 38–39
    ingredients to avoid, 39

uticaria, 82

vaccines, 17

vitamins, children and, 28

vomiting, 2

wheat allergy, 3, 4, 41–42, 52
    ingredients to avoid, 41–42
    wheat substitutes, 41, 42

wheezing, 2

Worcestershire sauce, 40